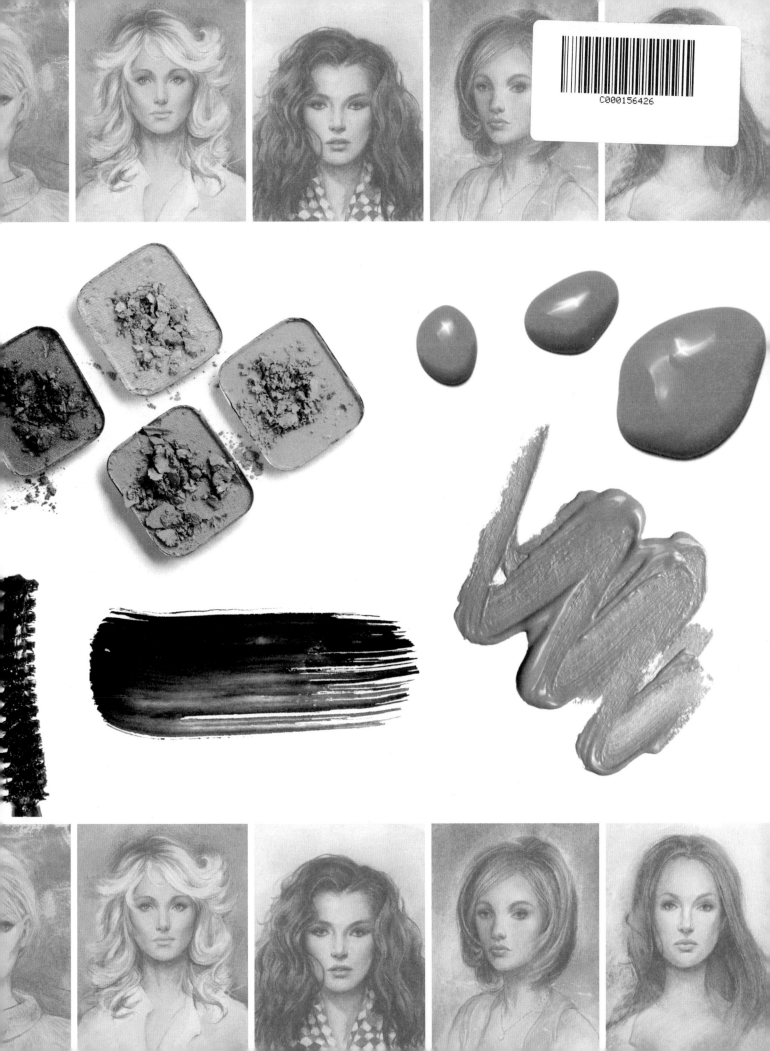

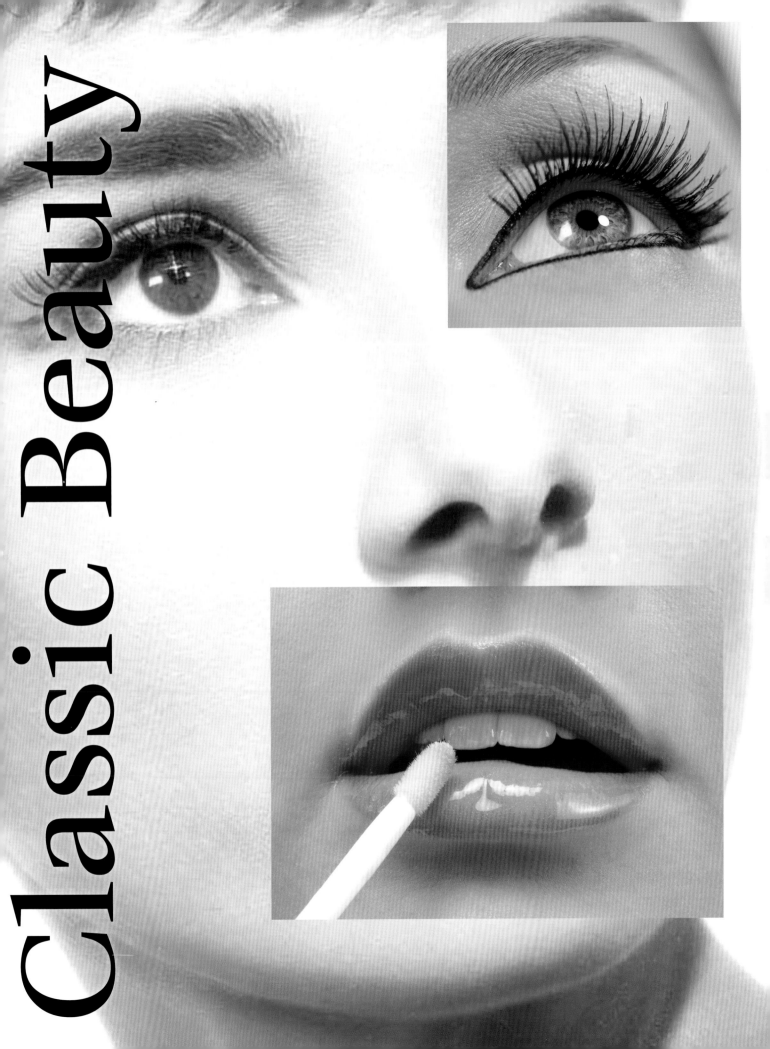

Classic Beauty

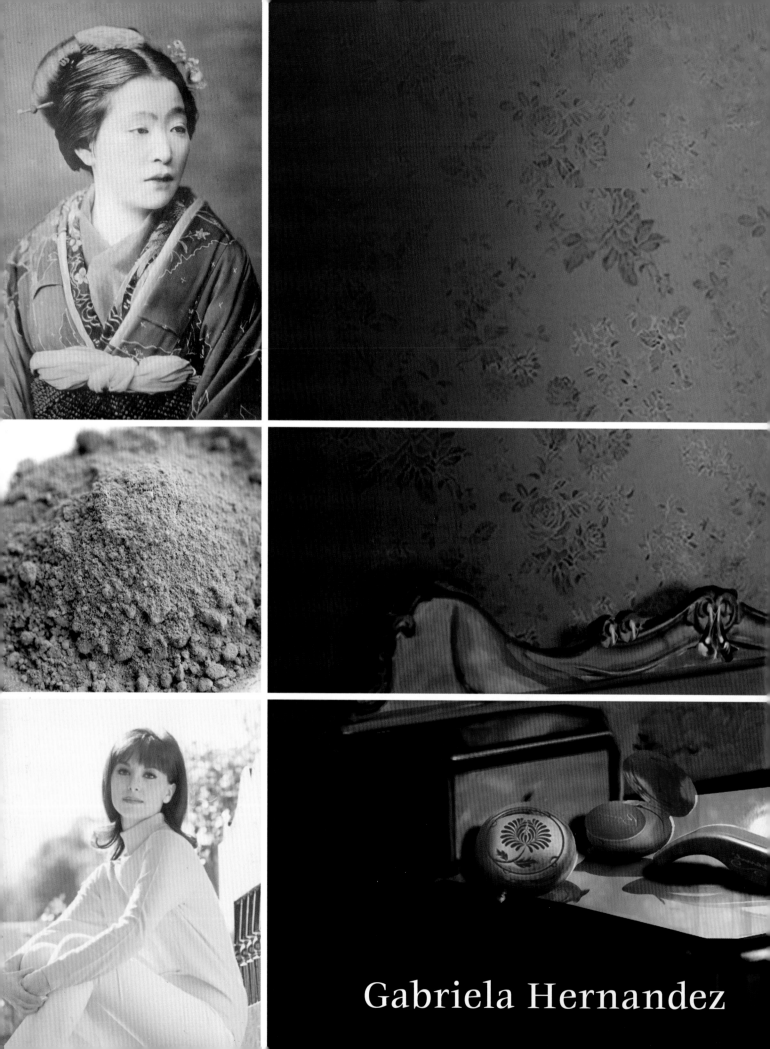

Gabriela Hernandez

Classic Beauty

The History of Makeup

2nd Edition

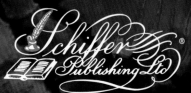

Schiffer
Publishing Ltd

4880 Lower Valley Road • Atglen, PA 19310

Disclaimers

This book presents beauty throughout history, breaking down the makeup styles for each decade while providing relevant background information that puts each look into perspective. The colors and techniques were gathered from many sources including period texts, history books, and actual samples of products. Every effort has been taken to provide accurate color and application technique information. Some information may be an approximation of accounts due to the lack of existing records from certain periods of time. Colors derived from actual samples may have suffered some alteration due to fading. Written accounts of similar colors vary depending on their source.

Please take precautions when attempting any of the looks described throughout this book. Most looks involve emphasizing specific parts of the face such as the eyebrows or the lips. Attempts should be done with a light hand to avoid looking theatrical, should that not be your intended use. Many looks involve excessive tweezing of the eyebrows or other hair on the face. Please be aware that eyebrow hair does not always grow back when shaved or tweezed. Use light and dark makeup or wax with spirit gum to simulate the intended effect without creating permanent changes to the face.

The ingredients listed for cosmetics from period texts may be harmful or poisonous. If you decide to purchase these items or try to create any of the recipes, do so at your own risk. Please research these ingredients before handling potentially harmful chemicals. Discontinue use of any substance that causes irritation to the skin.

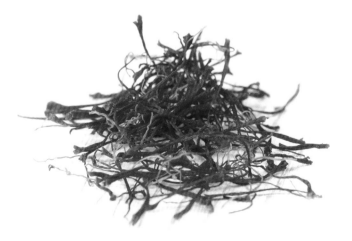

Other Schiffer Books on Related Subjects:
Permanent Makeup and Reconstructive Tattooing. Eleonora Habnit. ISBN: 0764318330. $29.95
Vintage Compacts & Beauty Accessories. Lynell Schwartz. ISBN: 0764301101. $34.95

Copyright © 2017 by Gabriela Hernandez

Library of Congress Control Number: 2016963722

Designed by John P. Cheek
Type set in Veljovic Medium/Aldine 721 BT

ISBN: 978-0-7643-5300-0
Printed in China

Schiffer Books are available at special discounts for bulk purchases for sales promotions or premiums. Special editions, including personalized covers, corporate imprints, and excerpts can be created in large quantities for special needs. For more information contact the publisher:

Published by Schiffer Publishing Ltd.
4880 Lower Valley Road
Atglen, PA 19310
Phone: (610) 593-1777; Fax: (610) 593-2002
E-mail: Info@schifferbooks.com

For the largest selection of fine reference books on this and related subjects, please visit our website at
www.schifferbooks.com
We are always looking for people to write books on new and related subjects. If you have an idea for a book please contact us at the above address.

This book may be purchased from the publisher.
Include $5.00 for shipping.
Please try your bookstore first.
You may write for a free catalog.

In Europe, Schiffer books are distributed by
Bushwood Books
6 Marksbury Ave.
Kew Gardens
Surrey TW9 4JF England
Phone: 44 (0) 20 8392 8585; Fax: 44 (0) 20 8392 9876
E-mail: info@bushwoodbooks.co.uk
Website: www.bushwoodbooks.co.uk

To my love and partner, Fergus, for his support and optimism.
Laugh and the world laughs with you.

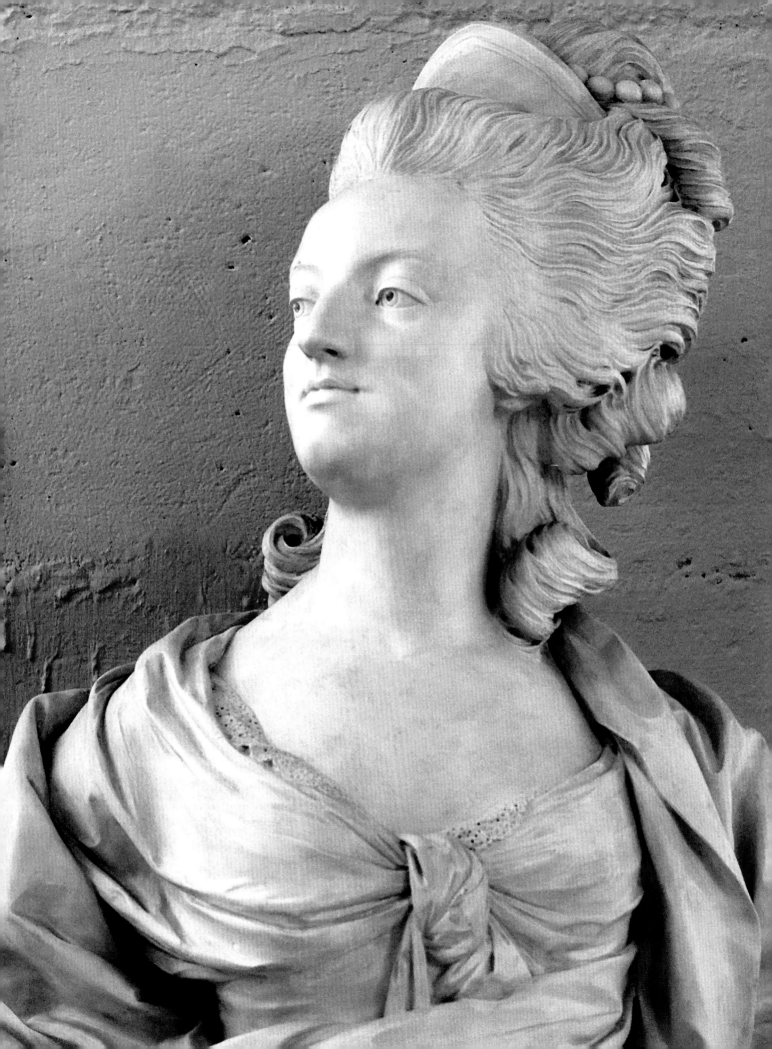

Contents

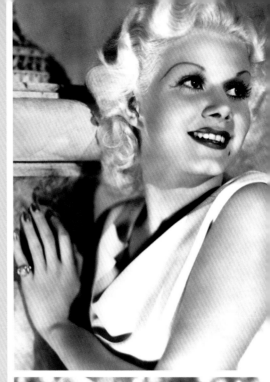

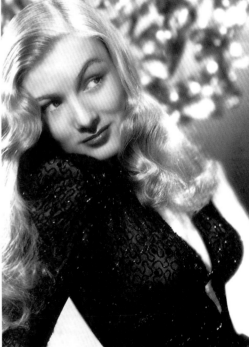

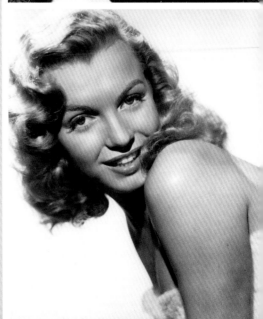

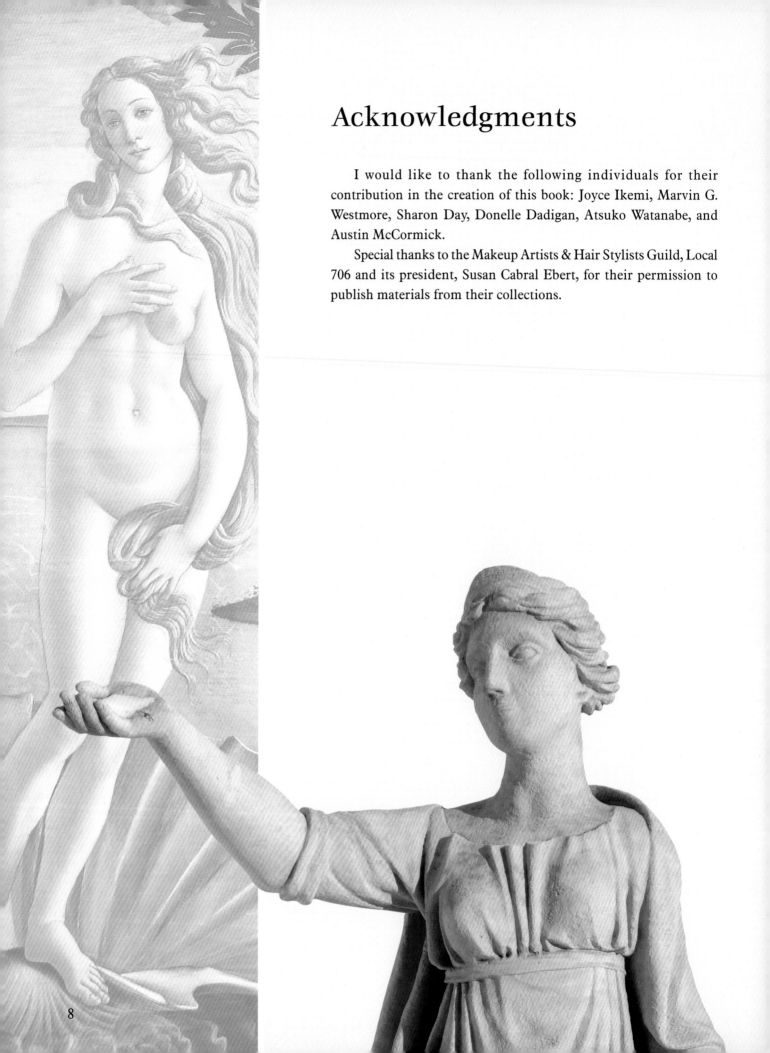

Acknowledgments

I would like to thank the following individuals for their contribution in the creation of this book: Joyce Ikemi, Marvin G. Westmore, Sharon Day, Donelle Dadigan, Atsuko Watanabe, and Austin McCormick.

Special thanks to the Makeup Artists & Hair Stylists Guild, Local 706 and its president, Susan Cabral Ebert, for their permission to publish materials from their collections.

8

Introduction

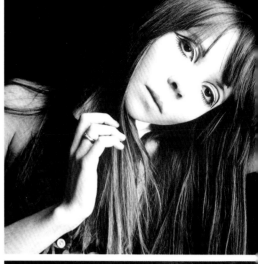

Beauty is in the eye of the beholder. While examining the origin of cosmetics for this book, this familiar phrase was found to describe more than just what each individual has defined physical beauty to be. Over the centuries, artists and writers interpreted what they characterized as beautiful through their paintings, sculptures, and prose. Specific looks were popularized, romanticized, and celebrated, bringing about ideal standards of beauty to be admired and imitated. Throughout the evolution of cosmetics, women have emulated the beautiful people seen within the arts and media, and cosmetic beauty aids have offered women the opportunity and confidence to achieve their utmost beauty potential. Because these standards have varied within each era's history, the concept of what defines beauty has changed and will always continue to do so.

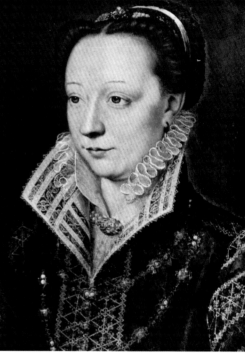

This book provides a grand tour of the rich history of facial trends and styles. The text shares a glimpse of each era from the political and social climates of the period and how these conditions were instrumental in molding the accepted beauty rituals of the time. Chapters that focus on specific decades give an overview of the changing face of beauty, photographs of prominent beauty icons, beauty facts, historical landmarks, reference guides, color palettes, and sample makeup routines of the period. The Product Development Timeline offers a look at the origins and inventions of cosmetics for the eyes, lips, and face.

Turn the page to begin an in-depth and historical journey of the many trends and styles of classic beauty looks throughout the ages.

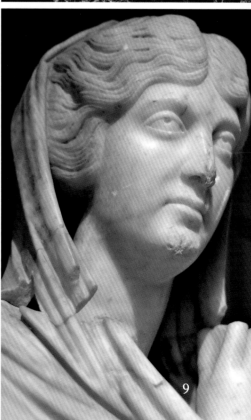

Historical TIMELINE
33,000 B.C. to A.D. 330

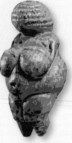

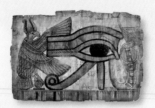

2500 B.C.
Cockleshells filled with colored pigments for eyes, lips, and cheeks are buried with their owners. Copper compounds create green and blue pigment. Iron oxides create red pigment. Manganese oxide creates black pigment. Burnt animal bone makes white pigment and lightens other colors.

25,000 B.C.
Fertility goddesses like the Venus of Willendorf shown here depict the power of female reproduction through massive curves.

5000 B.C.
Eye paint made from black galena and green malachite are the most commonly used cosmetics in Egypt.

4500 B.C.
The Japanese remove teeth and file them as a beauty ritual.

2000 B.C.
In Mesopotamia, oils and unguents infused with herbs are commonly used for bathing and body care.

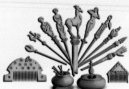

Toilet articles found at Pompeii. Bronze combs, hairpins made of ivory and gold.

15,000 B.C.
Pigments, such as manganese dioxides, are used in cave paintings and body painting, and used to color leather and wood. Colors include black, yellow, red, and ochre.

33,000 B.C.
Mineral pigments, such as ochre, are mixed with fat and used as sun block or protection from extreme weather. Rock paintings show figures adorned with stripes and dots for decoration. Body paints are used in ritual dances by aboriginal cultures.

3000 B.C.
Elaborately decorated razors and tweezers are used in grooming rituals.

1550 B.C.
In Crete, Greek women adorn elaborate hairstyles and apply rouge to the lips.

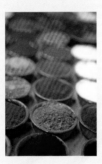

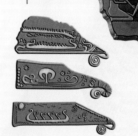

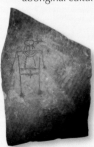

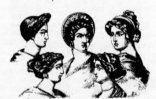

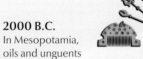

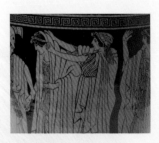

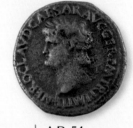

100 B.C.
The Greeks do not approve of cosmetics and stop their development. Manliness is in style. Men use oils and perfumes in public baths. Courtesans apply ceruse to whiten skin and scrape their skin clean with an ivory or metal blade.

A.D. 54
Poppaea, wife of the emperor of Rome Nero, uses white lead and chalk cake to whiten her complexion, Egyptian kohl for the lashes and eyelids, rouge, barley flour and butter to cure pimples, and pumice stones to whiten teeth. Coin of Nero.

A.D. 330
The Byzantine Empire, created from the remains of the Roman Empire, keeps open some of the trade routes for luxury goods.

400 B.C.
Greek vases depict young women at the toilette, and provide images of the ideal woman for others to follow. Boxes called pyxides store cosmetics, which include rouge made from alkanet, powder made from white lead, murex or vermillion, and kohl for the eyes.

The Ebers Papyrus, discovered by Georg Ebers in the nineteenth century, reveals a 110-page scroll of Egyptian medical texts. This work contains 700 formulas and remedies. The recipes are considered a mixture of science and magic with cures for most ailments.

550 B.C.
The Persians, in what is now Iran, import cosmetics from Egypt and use them liberally. Their love of luxury is shown in the use of jewelry, perfume, and intricate bathing practices.

129 B.C.
The Romans rule the civilized world. Their wealth opens up world trade, and leads to new discoveries in beauty enhancers and an emphasis on lightened hair. Hair is colored red or blonde with soap from Germany. Wigs are made from German hair. Vermillion is applied to the cheeks. Chalk powder is used to whiten skin. Statue of Latona, daughter of the Titans Coeus and Phoebe. Ancient Roman razor.

20 B.C.
Hair is colored with henna and bleached with lye to turn it red or gold. The early Church Fathers discourage the use of face paints.

A.D. 100
The Kama Sutra in India instructs women on how to tattoo and color their teeth, garments, hair, nails, and bodies.

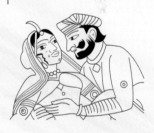

1450 B.C.
Glass containers for perfume, considered rare and precious, are found buried with the dead. Stone cosmetic palettes stained with green malachite or black galena are used to mix powder into a paste with water or oil and are applied with fingers or a wood applicator.

900 B.C.
Assyrians use elaborate cosmetic preparations to curl beards and style hair. Scented hair preparations containing beeswax and olive oil set the hair.

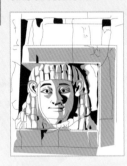

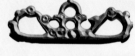

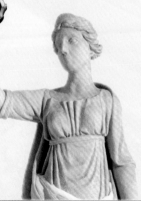

Opposite:
Colored pigments made
from ground minerals.

Stone wall with natural red
ochre.

The Origins of Cosmetics

The use of color on the face has been a ritual since the most primal of ages. Face paint was most likely used as a mask against evil figures and spirits rather than as a beauty enhancer. Primitive man lived in fear of the unknown and believed everything around him was hostile. Disguising himself with paint to appear fierce or unrecognizable gave him an advantage over his enemies. Face paint was not used amongst the women who stayed in the protected confines of their village.

Around 33,000 B.C., the use of face paint later developed into personal adornment and also as a skin protectant. The earliest pigments used were mineral oxide ochre powders and lampblack, the black soot collected from the smoke of carbon materials. A mixture of these pigments combined with animal fats made an effective blocking agent from the blazing sun and harsh winter winds. Ancient rock paintings show stylized figures adorned with distinctive stripes and dots. These designs decorated the body for ritual dance ceremonies before hunting or other significant events. Theories suggest that these ancestral humans gradually grew accustomed to the use of cosmetics for adornment as the practice of face painting became more habitual.

Pigments were discovered in the Lascaux caves of France dating back to 15,000 B.C. Among those found was manganese dioxide, a dense black color later used by the Egyptians for cosmetic purposes. Early pigments fell into three main colors represented in stable, vivid shades of black, yellow, and red. Prehistoric burials show the use of red ochre, an earthy iron oxide, on the body to prepare it for the afterlife. This reddish pigment was also prized as a colorant for leather, bone, and wood. Fragrant spices were also buried with the dead, as well as beads and seashells used as ornamentation.

We do not know the names of the formidable fertility goddesses of prehistory. The Venus of Willendorf, the most famous of these, does not even have a face. But her power, expressed in massive breasts and hips, is clearly felt. In fact, the power of these fertility goddesses, whose images may be found from the Americas to Africa to Asia, surpasses mere conception and gestation. Their power is the very self-renewing capacity of the cosmos.

The 5300-year-old remains of a Tyrolean man revealed the use of acupuncture and the art of tattooing to create permanent patterns on the skin.

In late prehistoric times, the practice of burning scented barks, seeds, and herbs in stone dishes may have been done to mask the stench of decaying flesh within burial tombs.

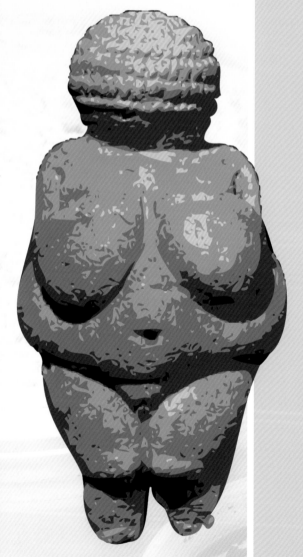

Venus of Willendorf, pre-historic fertility
sculpture, 30,000 – 25,000 B.C.

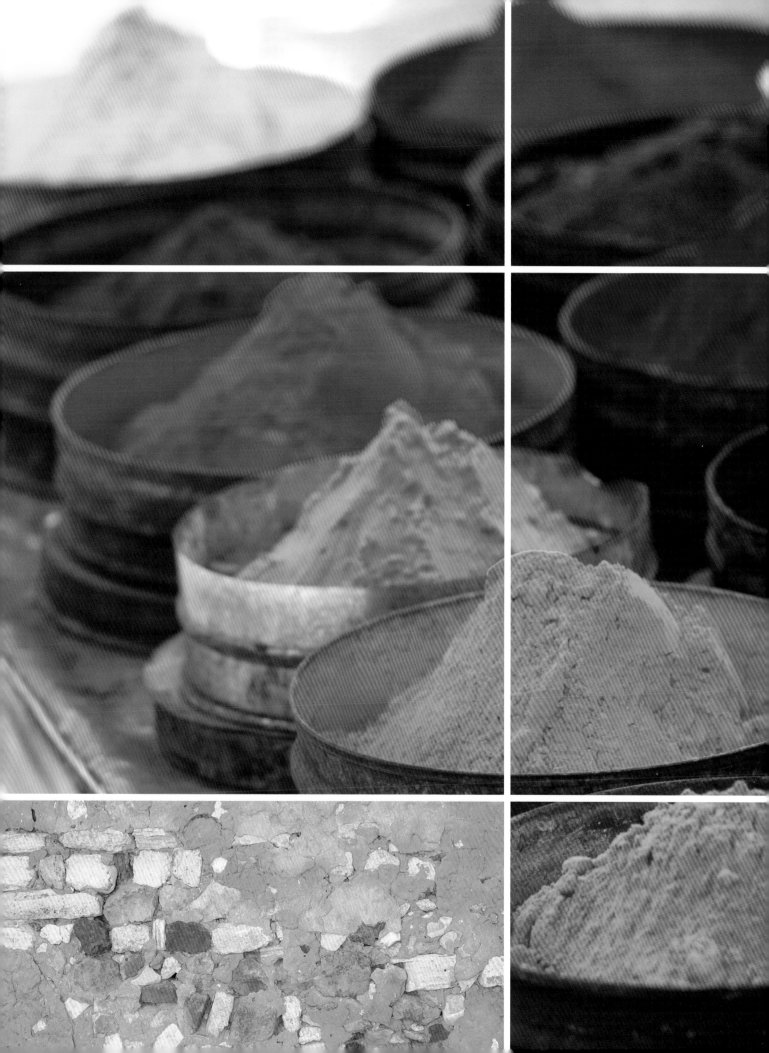

During the Bronze Age, razors and tweezers were used in grooming. These tools were often decorated with images of sailing vessels or the sun. Production of such items was facilitated through world trade, along with evolving trends in fashion and style ideas. This process flourished with the relentless Roman conquest of surrounding lands. Skilled Roman artisans who catered to the increasingly cosmopolitan tastes of the Roman ruling class seamlessly assimilated materials, design motifs, and cultural ideas from remote Viking territories and Asian civilizations.

Found artifacts, such as mirrors and other objects of adornment, suggest that a preoccupation with appearance has been present at all periods throughout history.

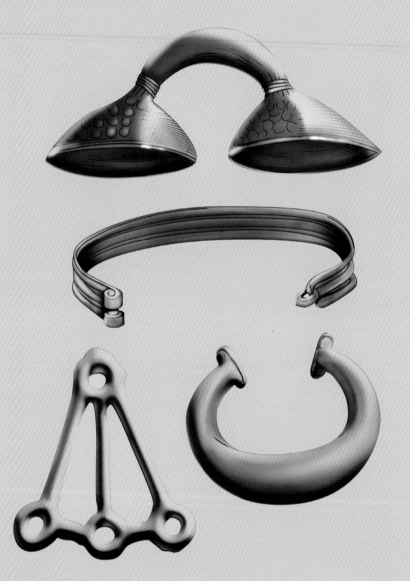

Ornamentations in gold and bronze, Bronze Age.

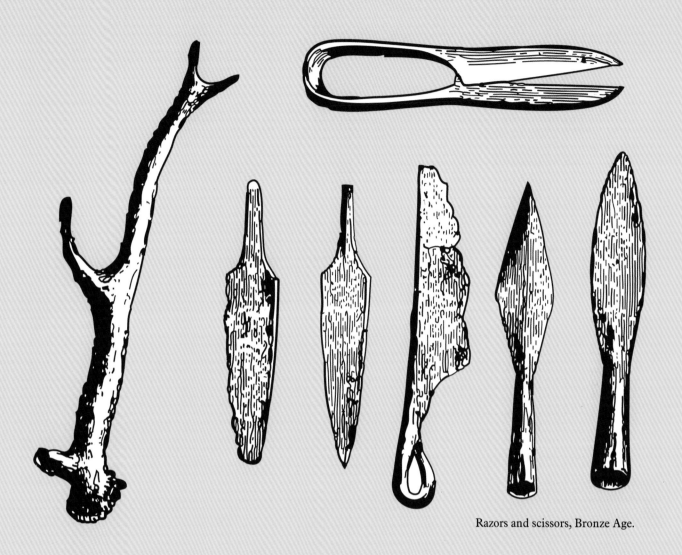

Razors and scissors, Bronze Age.

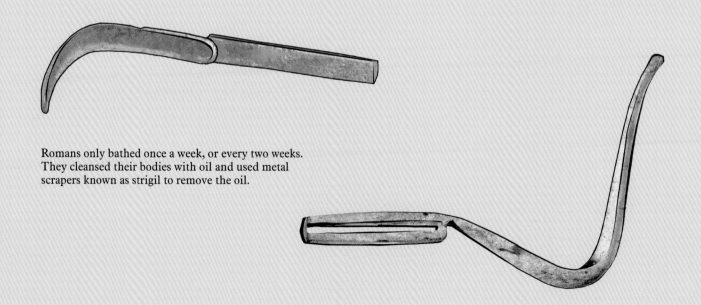

Romans only bathed once a week, or every two weeks.
They cleansed their bodies with oil and used metal
scrapers known as strigil to remove the oil.

15

Cosmetics in Antiquity

Egypt

Egypt developed as a civilization from 2659 B.C. to 1070 B.C. The Egyptians' use of cosmetics has been documented in detailed wall paintings and numerous artifacts. Their preoccupation with the care of the body was due to their belief in the union of the physical and the spiritual sides of life. They left significant compilations of medical texts, containing over 700 formulas and remedies for grooming and health care. The Ebers Papyrus, written in 1550 B.C. and translated by Georg Ebers in the late nineteenth century, gives insight into how the Egyptians mixed practical preparations with their magical beliefs.

The toilette box of a wealthy Egyptian woman often contained pumice stones, eye paint applicators, mineral powder, palettes to mix colors, and containers of colored powder. These included the green mineral malachite, red ochre used as a rouge and lip colorant, and black powder eyeliner known as kohl made from soot, galena, and other ingredients.

Bathing and personal cleanliness were of great importance to the Egyptians. They used sand mixed with clay and ash as an exfoliating scrub. Face masks of egg and scented oil were used to protect the skin from the drying sun and also as an insect repellent.

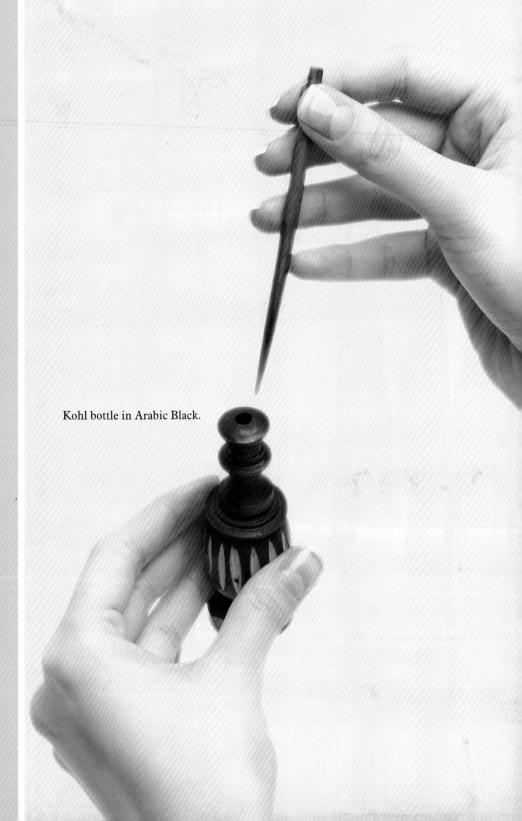

Kohl bottle in Arabic Black.

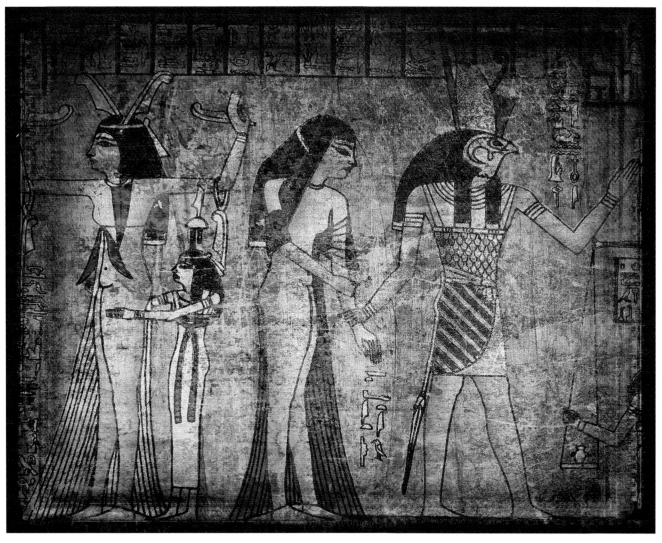

Ancient Egyptian papyrus.

Mineral galena in natural form.

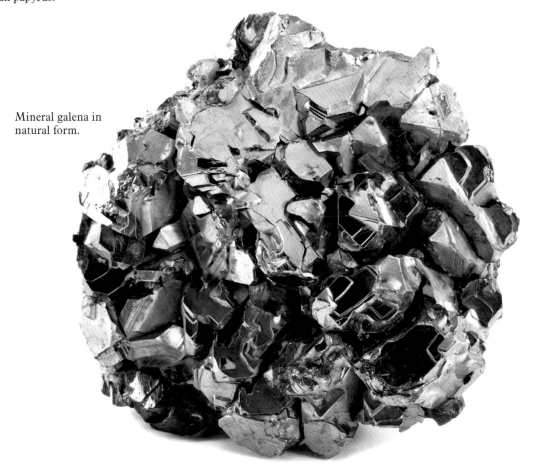

Anti-wrinkle creams, popular 3000 years ago, used frankincense as a soothing anti-inflammatory oil. These early wrinkle potions contained resin, wax, and oils to help the skin retain its moisture.

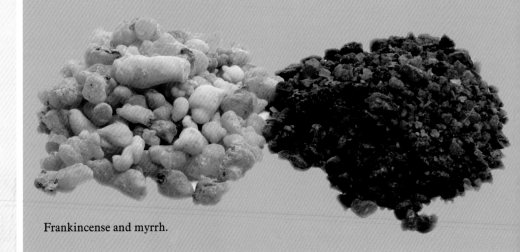

Frankincense and myrrh.

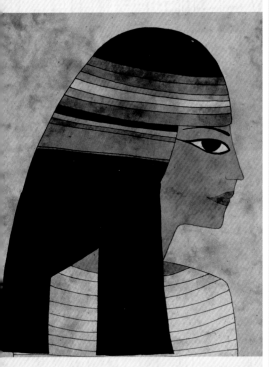

Ancient Egyptian woman collage.

The culture of ancient Egypt was deeply invested in the well-developed concept of the afterlife and immortality. The departed wore full makeup, as well as their best ceremonial finery into the next realm. Preservatives including frankincense and myrrh were used in the fastidious mummification process.

Kohl, green eye paint made from malachite, and red ochre used for rouge and lip color were the most popular forms of cosmetics for the common Egyptian woman.

Mesopotamia, now located in modern-day Iraq, was an ancient region of southwest Asia located between the Tigris and Euphrates rivers. Several of its early civilizations including tribes from Sumer, Akkad, Babylonia, and Assyria participated extensively in the trading of fashion and luxury goods. Historical evidence has revealed that around 2000 B.C., bathing and shaving were practiced, with the use of oils and salves. Oil was used daily to protect the skin from the harsh drying effects of the sun. Unguent and incense were prepared for use in the temples, and scented wax was used on the body as perfume for special occasions and celebrations. Palaces dedicated entire rooms to the blending of perfume.

From 2200 to 2177 B.C., Assyrian recipes for hair dyes were composed of cassia and leek extracts. Bas-reliefs from this period illustrated men with elaborate curled beards, which were groomed with the use of hairdressing pomades. These styling aids were made from olive oil, beeswax, and resins, and scented with barks and herbs.

Around 2500 B.C., the Babylonians used eye, cheek, and lip cosmetics. They filled shells with purple, red, yellow, blue, green, and black colored pigments. The pigments were lightened with the addition of burnt animal bone. Green eye paint was valued not only for its decorative purposes, but also as a sun protectant and as a medicinal ointment for eye infections.

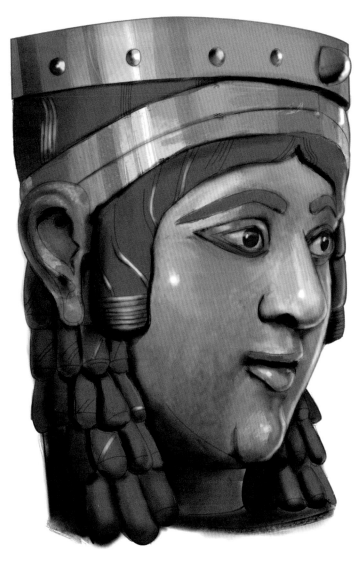

Neo-Assyrian head of woman, ruins in Nimrud, in ivory.

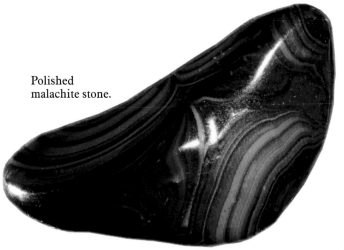

Polished malachite stone.

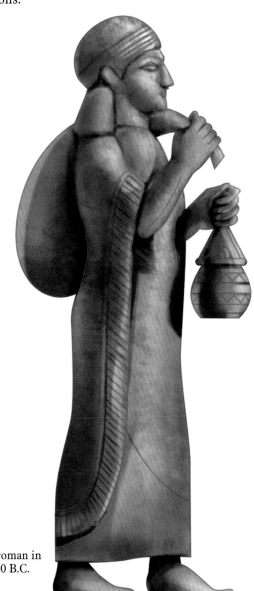

Assyrian working woman in traditional dress, 700 B.C.

Greece

The Greeks valued simplicity in facial adornment, but favored the use of perfumed oil. They developed unique methods for making perfume by using liquid tinting dyes. They preferred single note fragrances such as sage and rose.

Greek women adorned their hairstyles with ribbons and metal bands. Popular styles ranged from parted and smooth with ringlets, to the use of fancy ribbons and bandeaus. Hair oil was used to style the curls and was arranged high on the crown of the head.

The rest of the body was kept smooth and hairless with the use of tweezers and depilatories made with resinor plaster. The face was touched with rouge on the cheeks and lips. Some wall paintings show other markings on the face, including rows of dots and lines.

A Greek society woman was frequently shown in artwork holding a mirror as a reminder that she was an object of display who was expected to conform to the ideal.

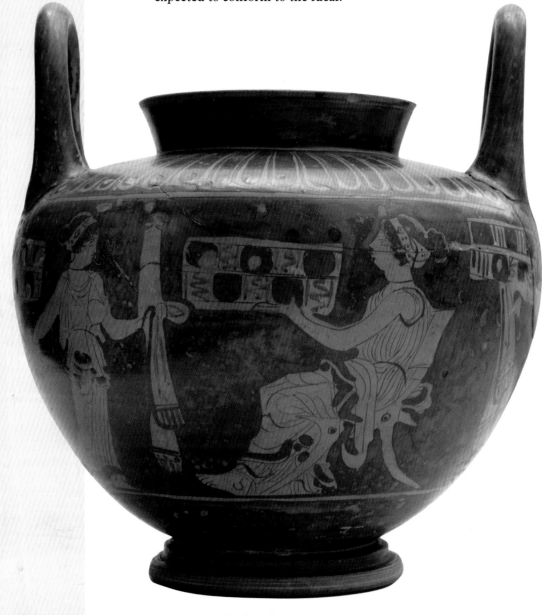

Ancient Greek vase.

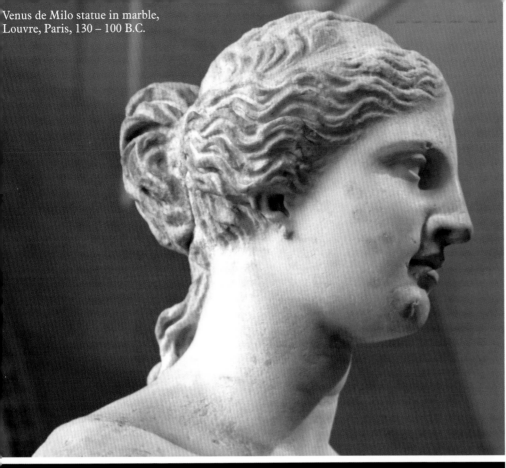

Venus de Milo statue in marble, Louvre, Paris, 130 – 100 B.C.

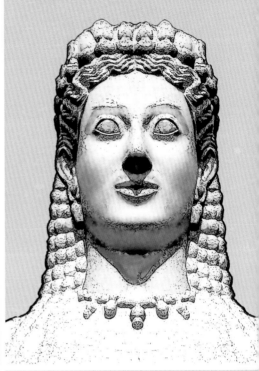

Greek kore statue with very ornate hairstyle. May represent a goddess, such as Persephone, priestess, or votary of a goddess.

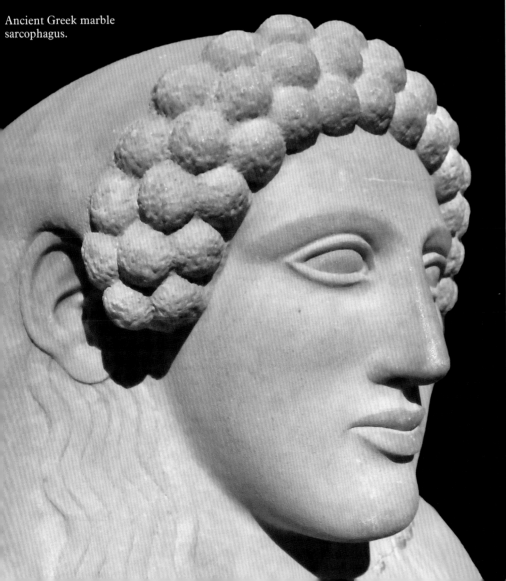

Ancient Greek marble sarcophagus.

Persia

Ancient Persian relief sculptures showed luxurious dresses and detailed grooming on the figures. Scented oil and cosmetics were sent regularly from Egypt packaged in small stone jars. Men used kohl around the eyes, a practice continued by Middle Eastern men today. They used ointment and perfume frequently to eliminate dirt and bad odors.

The Persians represented a transition between the ancient civilizations and the more classical Greeks and Romans. They embraced cosmetic practices that clearly influenced subsequent cultures.

21

Rome

The Romans wore rose red or pink tinted lip paint, eyeliner, darkened their eyebrows, and wore their hair curled with ribbons and pins. Chalk and vinegar face creams lightened the complexion. Finely ground orris root was used in face powder. The Roman woman favored skin cream and scented water as part of her toilette. Glass bottles with perfume and other unguents were found in Roman graves in A.D. 100 to 120.

Wealthy Roman women enlisted cosmetic artists and hair stylists to help with their beauty regimen. The cosmetic artist was called the cosmatae, and the mistress of the toilette, the ornatrix.

Classic Roman statue of Cornelia Antonia, in marble, A.D. 150.

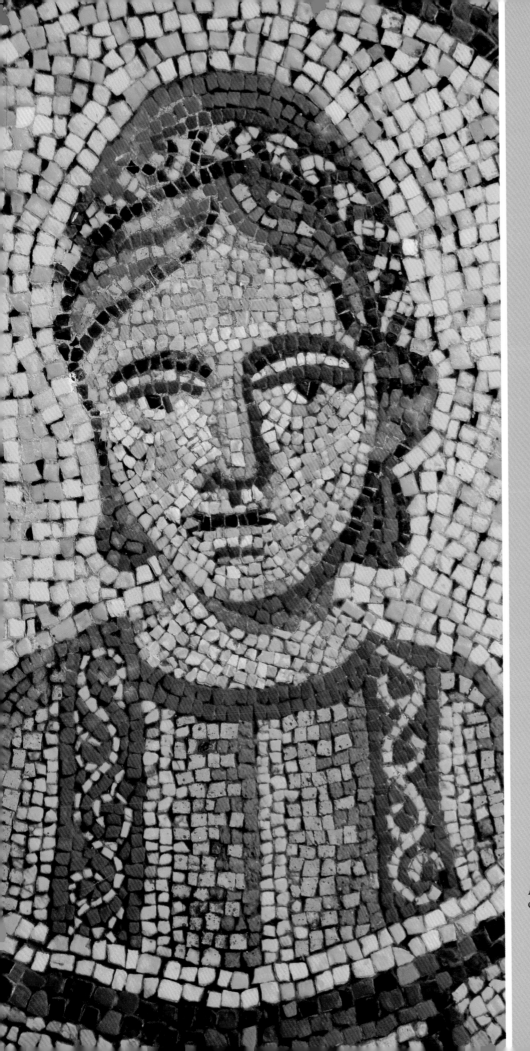

Ancient Roman mosaic
of a woman.

Historical TIMELINE
A.D. 330 to A.D. 1550

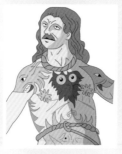

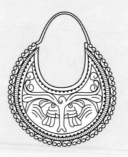

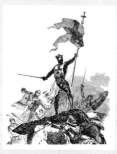

A.D. 900
Bleached hair, elaborate moustaches, and colorful tattoos are worn by Norse, Saxon, and Teuton warriors.

A.D. 1000
The Byzantines use rock-crystal cosmetic jars with jeweled lids. Crescent shaped pendants contain fragrance and are suspended from the ears.

The Crusades bring hair dye into fashion. Blonde or black are the preferred shades. Red hair has connotations of prostitution and witchcraft.

A.D. 700
The Norse, Saxons, and Teutons bring in the Dark Ages. Barbarians apply crude tattoos, pierce their ears, and wear heavy gold jewelry.

A.D. 950
Vikings bring aromatics to Europe from the Arab world via their ships and extensive trading routes.

Christianity puts an end to the inclusion of grave goods and promotes the care of the soul and not the physical body. The Old Testament mentions perfume and anointing oil. Church fathers promote the avoidance of such luxuries.

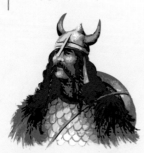

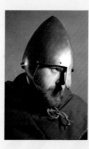

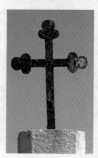

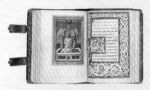

1400
Religious writers condemn any use of cosmetic products. Cosmetics are still in use by the upper class.

1470
Throughout the reign of Edward IV of England, cosmetics are applied by men and women. Standard products include whitening powder for the face, red salve for the lips, and kohl for the eyes and brows.

1550
Upper class women who could escape censure from the church continue to wear cosmetics. Beauty potions are linked to magic and incantations.

1482
The Birth of Venus by Botticelli. Both the kings of France and England have effeminate traits and wear cosmetics liberally.

1200
Jewish traders circulate spices, dyes, ointments, and perfumes after the Crusades.

1460
The ideal medieval face is pale and round with plucked eyebrows and a receding plucked hairline. The lips are small and the eyes pop as the only color on the face.

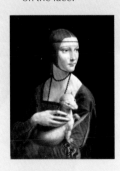

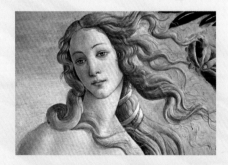

The Medieval Period

With the onset of Christianity, harsh weather conditions, and the spread of illness, cosmetics use was kept to a minimum throughout the Medieval period. Christian missionaries spurred a return to herbal potions and ointments for non-cosmetics use due to their belief that vanity was considered evil. Herbal preparations were used to clean and freshen the home and get rid of pests.

The year A.D. 1000 was significant in men's grooming practices. Many believed the anniversary of Christ's birth would bring about his return. Many men interpreted the scripture as saying it condemned the grooming of a man's hair. Shaving was stopped, and hair on the head grew wild and unruly. After the date passed, many followers believed they were saved and continued to grow their hair.

The church looked down upon bathing because the old Roman practice of communal baths were thought to promote promiscuity. Christians were scandalized by the discovery of ruins of Roman baths and brothels, where sexual scenes were depicted in mosaics, frescoes, and ceramics with wild abandon.

Information on hairstyles is limited due to the fact that most women wore their hair covered, although blond hair with abundant curls has been noted to be the preferred color and style. Both women and men used tweezers and combs for grooming.

The Norse, Teutons, and Saxons wore tattoos and heavy jewelry. They favored luxurious hair and produced finely carved combs to brush the hair and keep it clean of lice. Women used oils and pomades for the hair and herbs to freshen and soothe the skin. The Vikings continued to use the old Roman trading routes to supply the British with cosmetic goods.

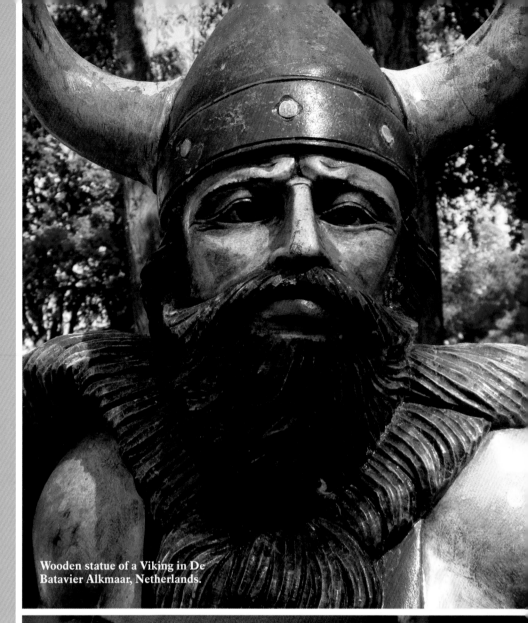

Wooden statue of a Viking in De Batavier Alkmaar, Netherlands.

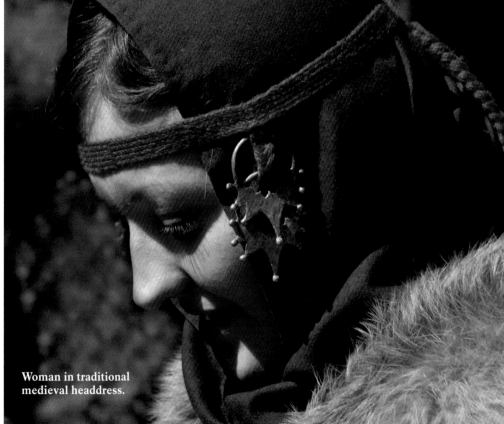

Woman in traditional medieval headdress.

The Middle Ages

The Crusades put rural European soldiers into contact with the sophisticated design technologies and decorative traditions of the fabled East.

During the Middle Ages, the Crusades introduced the worlds of fashion and cosmetics to English and European knights. These men witnessed new and exotic grooming customs and brought back their discoveries to the women at home. Trade with the East brought silk, gems, ivory, tea, coffee, and opium, as well as many spices, oils, and cosmetic ingredients to Europe, creating the need for alchemists to concoct potions and perfumes.

Arabian influences slowly came into European fashion through the use of hair dyes, lotions, and creams. Jewish spiritual healers mixed exotic beauty potions with ingredients imported from the Arab world. Women powdered their faces with flour and used harsh natural bleaches, such as lye, to get rid of freckles.

Although medieval life centered around wars and politics, there was still a taste for luxury goods and fineries within royal households. Both men and women of the royal court kept dedicated barbers and cosmeticians at hand.

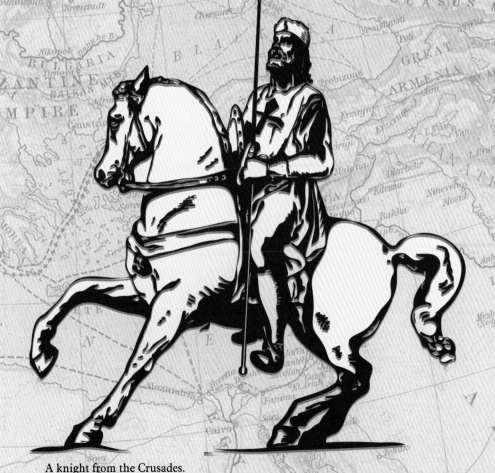

A knight from the Crusades.

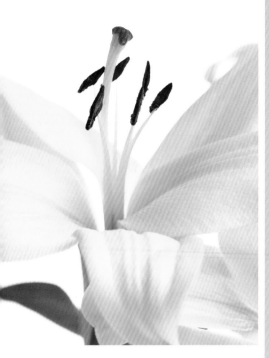

White lily.

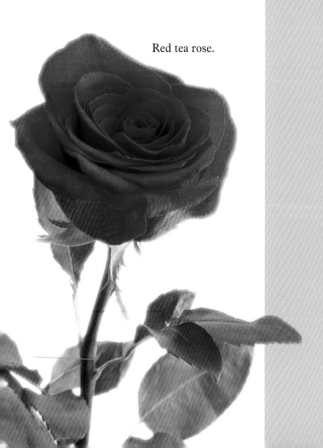

Red tea rose.

Elizabeth Woodville, queen and consort of King Edward IV of England, was regarded as the ideal beauty of the time. She had a high forehead with an oval face, light hair, straight nose, and small lips.

The courtesans of the fifteenth century wore their cosmetics liberally. They were characterized by heavily painted faces, elaborate wigs, and high-stacked shoes called pianelles.

Toiletry kits of the era included toothpicks, tweezers, ear scoops, small mirrors, and combs made from wood, bone, or horn. Many of these items were similar to the ones found in Rome.

The lily and the rose, emblematic symbols of chivalry, also represented the ideal colors of beauty. A white lily represented a pale complexion and a red rose represented the color of youthful lips. These flowers also represented the secretive, symbolic irony of courtly love: white for the noble lady's steadfast chastity and red for her knight's carnal passion.

Perfumed waters and other scented fluids were commonly used to clean and freshen up the home. Cleansing herbs contained antibacterial properties, which protected against infectious diseases. Popular perfumes were made from violet flowers that were pressed and mixed with purified lard.

As information crossed the Channel regularly, French fashions slowly began to influence the courts in Britain. The use of pomanders to scent dresses originated in France. Regular bathing and cleanliness was practiced using large sponges and basins of water sprinkled with fresh herbs and flowers. The commoners used communal tubs and public baths. The pestilence of 1348 and the Black Plague forced many of these establishments to close. These factors marked a return to a simpler lifestyle, one that did not include cosmetic niceties.

By the end of the Middle Ages, women benefited from new trade and cultural exchanges. Paint, soap, mirrors, dyes, and perfumes became easily available. The use of these products was recognized, but not consumed by all for economic or religious reasons.

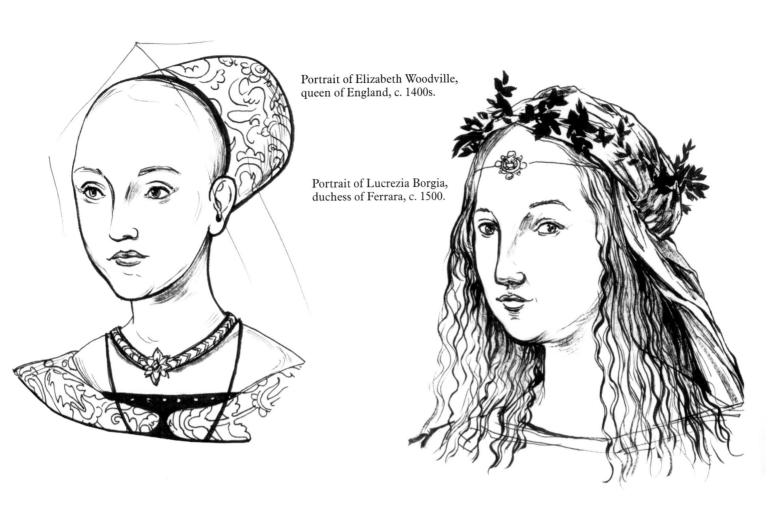

Portrait of Elizabeth Woodville, queen of England, c. 1400s.

Portrait of Lucrezia Borgia, duchess of Ferrara, c. 1500.

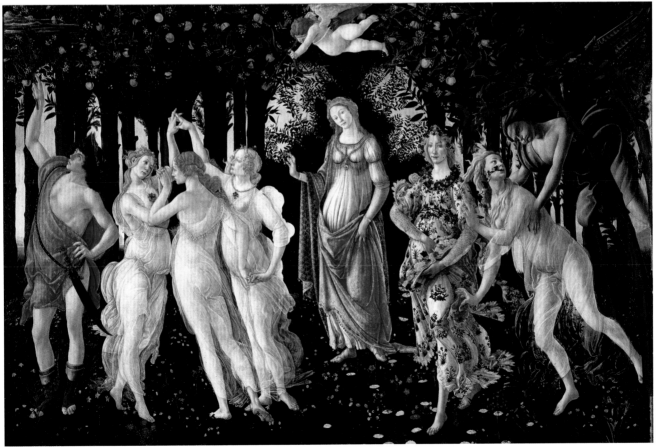

Primavera by Boticelli, 1482.

Historical TIMELINE
A.D. 1600 to A.D. 1789

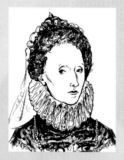

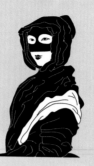

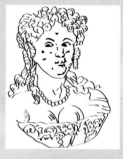

1630
Queen Elizabeth I makes cosmetics use acceptable among elegant women. The French's use of cosmetics increases to the point where even nuns curl and powder their hair. Working class women apply flour as white powder to the face.

1643
Women use cutout leather masks when outdoors to protect skin from the sun and also as a partial disguise for flirtation.

1660
Charles II substitutes a wig for his own hair and starts the trend of cutting the hair short or shaving it off. Men as well as women practice these trends.

1720
Enamel, rouge, white powder, and masks are used in England to distinguish the upper class in court society. Patches to cover pimples are given different names and meanings depending on their placement on the face.

1640
Eskimo tribes paint their faces blue and yellow to the surprise of early European explorers.

1600
Beauty looks to Venice as a supplier of cosmetic goods, including the deadly lead-based ceruse.

1653
Restoration women are very plain. The law punishes excessive ornamentation. The forehead is exposed and the hair falls naturally to the sides.

1700
After witchcraft disappears and persecution subsides, sailors adopt tattooing. Tattoos are seen as good luck charms and status symbols.

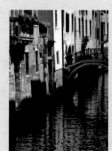

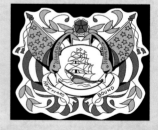

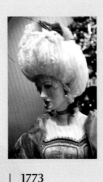

1773
Hair is set with lard, liberally dusted with white powder, and decorated with feathers and artificial flowers. The towering hairpieces are often infested with mice and fleas. Cages made of silver or gold wire protect the wigs while not in use.

1786
England imposes a heavy tax on cosmetics. A license is required for their sale in shops. Beauty preparations become more costly, prompting many women to follow home recipes from women's magazines.

Women wear masks made of black silk or velvet-covered leather as a tool for seduction. This explains the unimportance of eye makeup during the period. The standard colors used on the face are white ceruse and Spanish red.

Perfume is used lavishly to mask odors and dirt, since bathing is not a popular ritual, and the elaborate clothing is impossible to clean.

1770
Lipsticks, which resemble chalks, are made from ground plaster of Paris and carmine or vegetable dyes added for coloring.

Male members of the traveling elite form the Macaroni Club. These men wear Italian fashions, long curled hairdos, heavy makeup, and are ridiculed for their excessive preoccupation with fashion. They are mentioned in the popular song *Yankee Doodle.*

1789
The French Revolution marks the end of the aristocratic society in France and an end to the extremely artificial look. Cosmetic face paints are considered vulgar. People spend time in the country and adopt a natural look. Hair is cut short for men and white powder is abandoned.

1760
England's smallpox epidemic and the usage of ceruse for whitening the skin leaves many with permanently scarred and pitted complexions. Patches of cloth or leather, some shaped like stars and moons, hide scars.

1750
France produces the most popular cosmetics of the time, including cakes of lip salve, boxes of pomatum, and perfumed ointment. They are sent back to Britain by travelers. In America, women use similar preparations in a more moderate manner, and keep their looks more natural. Portrait of Hortense Mancini, duchess of Mazarin.

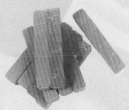

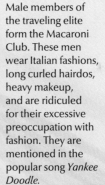

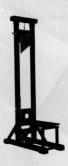

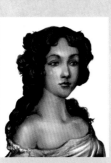

Sixteenth and Seventeenth Centuries

The House of Tudor and the reign of Queen Elizabeth I of England, "The Virgin Queen," brought prosperity and a new appreciation for the cosmetic arts. The members of Elizabeth's court used cosmetics such as white lead powder, Spanish red rouge, and hair dye on a regular basis.

Queen Elizabeth's porcelain white look remained popular until the 1800s. The use of white lead powder, or ceruse, created her white matte complexion and she reportedly shaved or plucked her hairline to make her already high forehead seem even higher, further asserting her refinement and aristocracy.

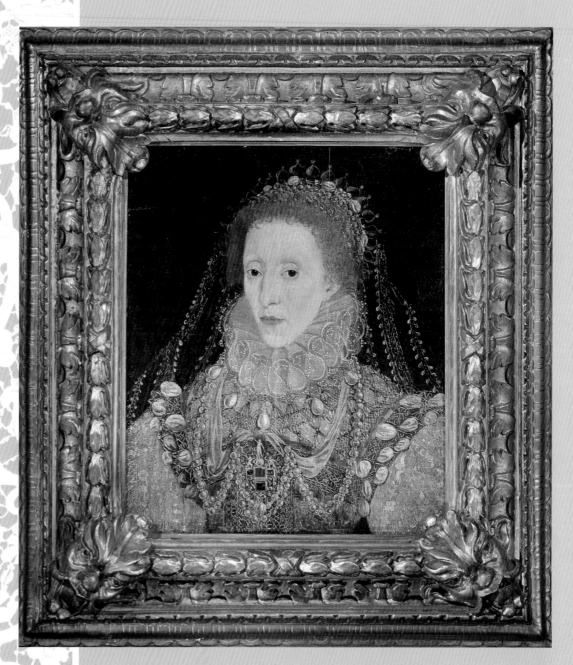

Portrait of Queen Elizabeth I of England.

Venice, the undisputed center of fashion at the time, was the main exporter of ceruse. Although very poisonous, ceruse was one of the most expensive cosmetic treatments favored by the wealthier classes. To make the skin seem translucent, veins were painted on the neck and chest. Cheeks and lips were bright pink and stood out against one's ghostly white complexion.

Men and women belonging to court circles carried mirrors made of glass or steel. They applied heavy musky scents to clothing and gloves as opposed to directly on the skin. They wore patches on the face to cover scars and pockmarks. The perfumes of the period were extremely pungent. When a 1590 Elizabethan prayer book was discovered over 400 years later, it still maintained a trace of musk.

Hair was commonly dyed auburn during the reign of Elizabeth, but blonde remained the most popular shade of hair color. The potions used to lighten the hair were made with rhubarb steeped with wine or lye. This would leave hair a golden shade, but in poor condition. A safer dye, which colored the hair a dark blonde, was made with turmeric and alum.

The expansion of trade and the founding of the East India Company in the seventeenth century brought exotic spices and scents to Britain. Fashion trends filtered down to the lower classes as many homes contained warm chambers to dry herbs and brew home recipes. Medicinal recipes were adapted into cosmetic uses. Herb vinegars used to ward off disease were turned into fragrant waters to freshen up clothing and the home. Books on the preparation of cosmetic aids flourished, with many detailing the art of adornment.

The Puritan influences of the time created differences in opinion about the use of cosmetics amongst the varying social classes. Makeup was a controversial topic during this period. The Puritans believed cosmetics were a deceptive device to lure men into marriage. Cosmetics were tied to witchcraft, and its use ultimately became punishable by law. A pale, hairless face was the ideal standard of beauty among Puritan women, and they plucked their hair mercilessly to remove eyebrows and bare an extended forehead. The Puritans believed that the noble men and women who carried mirrors saw the devil in their own reflections.

Puritans did favor the use of soap, but were opposed to perfumed aromas, claiming they dulled the spirit and the senses. Beautification of any form was considered sinful, and there were many cautionary tales of women who paid the ultimate price of being taken by the devil after using beauty aids.

Paint and prostitution went hand in hand in the minds of the people. But beautification with cosmetic preparations, home made or purchased, was still practiced by many women, because looking beautiful opened the door to preferential treatment by men.

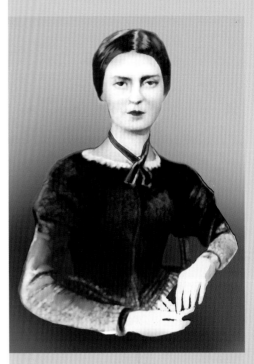

Decades later, poet Emily Dickinson (1830–1886) epitomized the austere Puritan psyche in Colonial America.

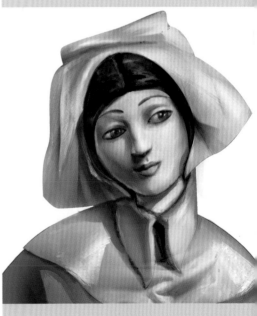

A seventeenth century Puritan woman.

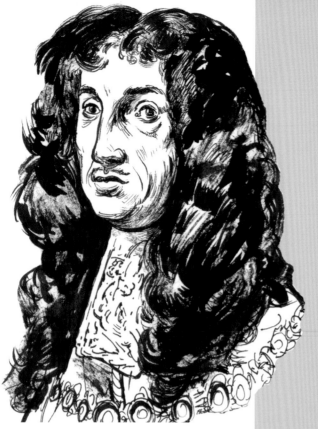

King Charles II of England.

The restoration of Charles II from 1660 to 1685 and the end of Puritan rule brought a much freer use of cosmetics and extravagance. Incense and soap were widely consumed by the wealthy.

Cosmetic crayons formulated with plaster, colorant, and wax were the equivalent of greasepaints. Pomanders became more elaborate and were joined by smelling boxes, ornate little boxes that could be carried and sniffed frequently to conceal bad odors. The latter could hold liquid scent or a scented cloth. Even clergymen used cosmetics in the form of aromatic vinegars and pomanders made from hollowed out oranges filled with lavender, rosemary, or clove.

As prices dropped, cosmetics were now available to the masses. Red ochre and powder could be obtained for a penny. Merchants, commoners, and peasants bought cosmetic preparations from peddlers. They sold ochre for the cheeks, dyes for the hair, cures for freckles, and other miracle creams. Most of these were ineffective formulas sold to a gullible clientele by sharp talking salesmen. It was the beginning of oral hygiene as teeth were cleaned with abrasive powder sweetened with honey or herbs. Toothpicks were used, and the mouth was rinsed with water. Sweets were not yet known to cause tooth decay.

A common list of toiletries used by women included bear's grease, orange flower water, perfumed oil, powder boxes, hair brushes, dressing pins, taffeta or leather face patches, and face paints.

Flower water was commonly used to bathe, but hot water was feared as possibly cooking the flesh. Many chose not to bathe and instead used a sponge soaked in perfume to mask bad odors.

Women used cleansing creams to treat their complexions. These were comprised of a mixture of soap and astringent ingredients that remained in use throughout the Victorian period.

Seventeenth century silver pomander/ vinaigrette box, 1695.

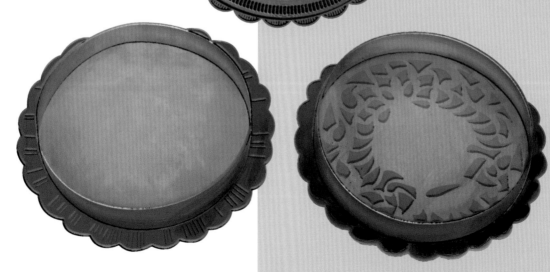

The Eighteenth Century

The eighteenth century was characterized by an exaggerated use of cosmetics amongst the European aristocracy. An interest in elaborate dress and high fashion separated the rich from the poor. The application of rouge was lavish in the royal courts, and powders and paints were used to create strong dramatic looks. The hair was styled in enormous towers, and perfume was heavily scented and applied in excess.

Queen Marie Antoinette of France practiced the ritual of a public toilette. An elaborate routine was carefully staged to allow favored members of the royal court to accompany her. In these public forums, women discussed many issues besides their looks and often invited intellectual guests to engage in conversation.

The significance of perfume was highlighted in France throughout the eighteenth century. Some of the largest perfume houses, such as Houbigant, established during the eighteenth century, are still in existence to this day. The court of Louis XV was nicknamed the

Sculpture of Marie Antoinette, c. 1750.

Engraving, Lafayette meets with Louis XVI and Marie Antoinette, 1859.

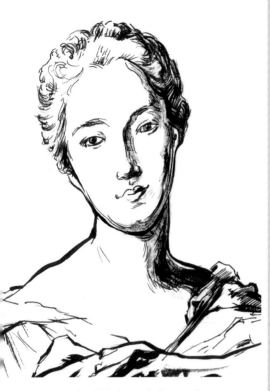

Portrait of Madame de Pompadour.

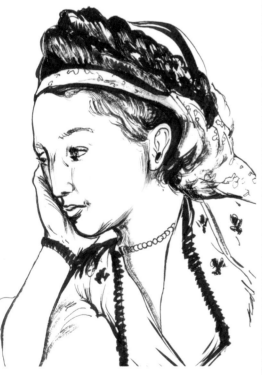

Portrait of Mary Gunning, countess of Coventry.

"perfumed court." King Louis' mistress, Madame de Pompadour, was credited with establishing the French cities of Montpellier and Grasse as centers of the perfume world. This is where the perfume making processes of enfleurage, maceration, and lavage made subtle delicate fragrances possible. Fragrance was sprinkled on items such as clothing, breath freshener pastilles, home incense, and potpourri. Fancy trinket boxes contained squares of fabric dipped in fragrance. In 1789, with the onset of the French Revolution, the use of perfume was banned in France as an unnecessary practice, but it made a return during Napoleon's reign.

Although people were fully aware of the poisonous and potentially fatal nature of the white powder ceruse, it remained a popular cosmetics item. It was commonly applied in thick layers, and keeping it on for long periods of time often hid the skin damage caused by its use. The excessive use of this poisonous cosmetic, in turn led to the early demise of many wealthy beauties. The Gunning sisters of Ireland gained notoriety in London for their ravishing good looks. Toxins accumulated from ceruse caused the death of one of the sisters in her early 20s, but this still did not hamper ceruse's use and popularity among beauty conscious individuals.

The eighteenth century was the age of beauty and materialism. For middle class women, enhancing one's looks with a careful application of cosmetics was an important step to securing a respectable marriage and high social status. Society women balanced between looking fashionable and not appearing overtly made up because obvious use of paint was looked down upon. With a disdain for royalty and nobility during the French Revolution, powdered curls gave way to more natural styles in the 1770s.

Cosmetic trends of the day called for rouge as its main facial focal point. Shades varied from pale pink to bright orange according to the changes in fashion. Rouge was the most accepted of the color cosmetics, being worn by both men and women. Men used Spanish pads of wool tinted with carmine to color the cheeks. The origin of the ingredients also imparted differences in rouge tints. Carmine made from insects created strong blue-red colors. Mineral-based pigments created orange-red colors. Vegetable-based rouges gave off more natural transparent red tones.

Cochineal, an insect collected in Mexico and imported back to Europe, was used to create a vivid crimson dye. Some accounts maintain that cochineal, which live in the prickly pear cactus, were used to dye the brilliant woolen uniforms of the famous British red coats. Cochineal is still used in lipstick formulations today.

Darker tones were preferred in France and not in Britain. Throughout Europe, cakes of lip salve, pomatum, and perfumed ointments became available in an array of formulas. Pale skin, black brows, and rose colored cheeks and lips comprised the facial makeup of the ideal face. Women's eyebrows were very defined and tinted with elderberry juice or darkened with burnt cork. False brows made from mouse hair were fashionable from 1700 to 1780.

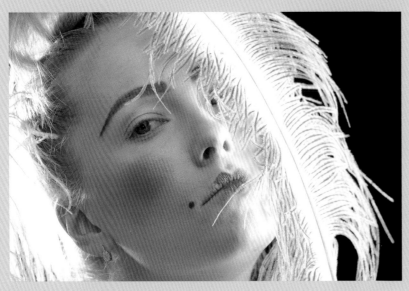

Bright rouge over white ceruse powder. Practiced by the middle class and nobility.

In America, people sported a more natural appearance and used paints sparingly. The macaroni, or British dandy in America, wore a large powdered wig, rouge and powder, and was extravagant in his use of fashion. He was often satirized for his unfitness for real work and his feminine practices.

For many people of the eighteenth century, dental hygiene was an overlooked grooming practice. Many individuals used cork "plumpers" to avoid hollow cheeks caused by tooth loss. False teeth were produced from bone or ivory. George Washington had a set of dentures made from animal teeth and ivory. Real teeth were occasionally extracted from corpses. Tooth powders were used as abrasives to clean teeth. Sponges and tongue scrapers that abated bad breath were used as popular teeth cleaners.

The first fashion magazines went into publication in the eighteenth century. They depicted fashion and hairstyle trends popular with vanity-seeking women of the day. In 1770, magazines like *The Lady's Magazine* provided limited details in its text and were published for women already familiar with fashionable looks. By the end of the century, Paris' *Journal de la Mode* was available in America and Britain, and broadened the business of fashion to a much wider audience.

In 1786, taxes were imposed on cosmetic articles in England. Special licenses were required to wear hair powder. Scented hair powder, pomade, and hairpieces were necessary to attain the enormous heights of the Rococo hairstyles, and no price was too high to pay for one to keep up with the popular styles of the time. Fines were eventually lifted by the 1800s when the hair powder trend subsided, and the only ones left wearing powders were the live-in servants of the wealthy.

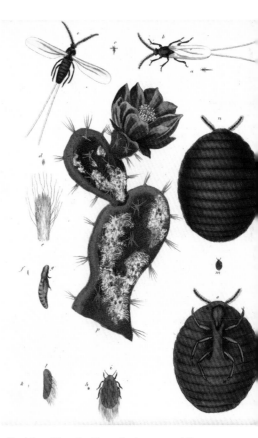

Cochineal beetle, *Dactylopius coccus* (*Coccus cacti*) on a prickly pear cactus, Opuntia species. Handcolored lithograph from Georg Friedrich Treitschke's Gallery of Natural History, *Naturhistorischer Bildersaal des Thierreiches*, Liepzig, 1840.

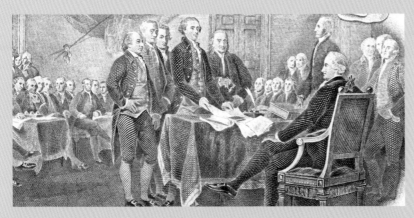

Popular hairstyles of the late eighteenth century in America.

Historical TIMELINE

A.D. 1800 to A.D. 1897

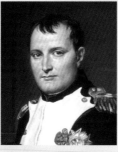

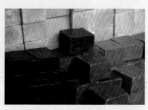

1804
Napoleon Bonaparte crowns himself Emperor of France and lifts the restriction of perfumers in Grasse installed by the French Revolution.

1825
The Art of Beauty is published anonymously. It suggests that cosmetic products are meant to improve the skin, not to hide flaws. It also suggests that bathing frequently and using a variety of ointments and lotions will enhance beauty.

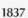

1837
Hair pomade, oil, cleanser, and dye are essential elements for grooming due in part to the popular ringlet curl hairstyles for men and women.

1850
The manufacture of soap becomes a thriving business in Victorian England with several factories including Yardley and Statham. English soap gains recognition for excellence and wins several medals at the Great Exhibition of 1851.

1806
Colgate and Company is founded by William Colgate.

1800
Beau Brummell embodies the new look in gentlemen's fashion with impeccable cleanliness and the use of delicate cologne. Two popular styles of cravats.

1830
Chinese Boxes are the first makeup palettes. They contain papers coated with black powder for eyebrows, red powder for cheeks, and white pearl powder for the face.

1842
During Queen Victoria's reign, an obsession with cleanliness brings about the establishment of public baths in Liverpool, England.

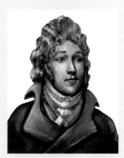

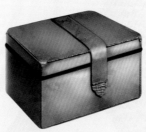

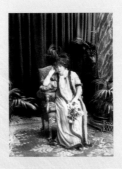
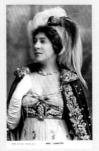
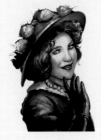

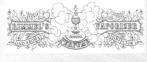

1851
Eugene Rimmel wins an honorable mention award for his perfume at the Great Exhibition. He later becomes famous in the cosmetics industry.

1870
France, England, and Portugal import many color cosmetics. The most popular are perfumes from France, lotions and soaps from England, and rouge dishes from Portugal.

1890
Sarah Bernhardt and Lillie Langtry create a new image of beauty by using kohl eye makeup and carmine lip coloring. Women begin to use cosmetics more liberally. Lampblack is used as a precursor to mascara.

1895
Julian Eltinge, female impersonator and stage actor, is so admired for his beauty that he markets and sells his own cosmetics line.

Jules Hauel, Roussel, and Bazin dominate perfume manufacturing in America.

1860
Dr. Gouraud's cosmetics and Jones's preparations are heavily advertised in the *New York Daily Tribune*. The main cities for cosmetics distribution are New York, Philadelphia, and Boston. Sales agents and traders sell products to smaller cities and towns.

1886
Mrs. Frances Hemming opens a salon in London and sells beauty preparations under the brand name of Cyclax.

The first academy of hairdressing is established with formal training and certification.

1897
Sears offers its own line of cosmetic products.

The Nineteenth Century

A more subtle use of cosmetics characterized the nineteenth century. With the coronation of Queen Victoria in England, she represented youthful modesty and brought with her the popularity of delicate toilette waters and pearl powders to gently lighten the complexion.

Heavy scents were unfavorable throughout Victorian fashion, but patchouli from India became popular because imported Kashmir shawls were packed with twigs of this scent to guard against moths. These fragranced shawls were in fashion throughout Victorian England.

During Victoria's reign and Britain's conquest of the Indian subcontinent, wearing Indian finery, including paisley and calico patterns was considered a gesture of nationalistic pride.

Victorian dressing sets were made of luxurious materials. They included combs, brushes, mirrors, nail buffers, hatpin trays, and jewelry boxes. With the overall acceptance of cosmetics and the fact that cosmetic goods were easily available to women by way of the European and American general stores, special attention was paid to impeccable grooming habits.

The Victorians believed in cleanliness, and washing became a daily ritual. They placed basins and small tubs in their bedrooms. Sanitation issues were problematic in English towns. The National Public Health Act in 1848 made it the law to have sanitary toilets in every home. Such toilets consisted mainly of a pit full of ashes. The installation of sewer systems also helped to alleviate sanitation issues.

Victorian balls demanded special toiletries and fashionable dresses. Dress guards and chemises or undergarments were laundered to absorb perspiration from dancing, but natural body odors were common and not considered offensive as they are today.

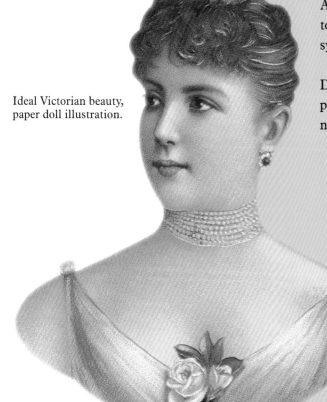

Portrait of Queen Victoria of England, from the Opening of the Crystal Palace.

Ideal Victorian beauty, paper doll illustration.

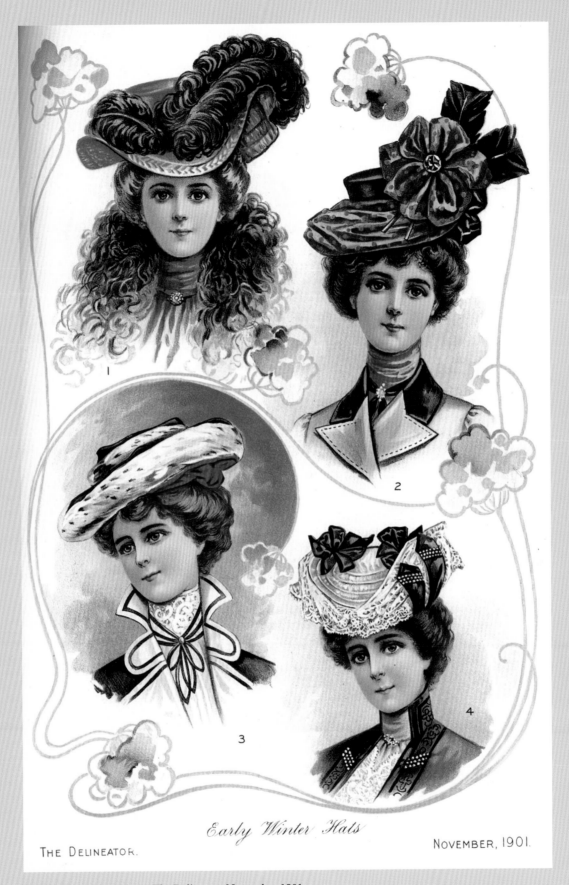

Early Winter Hats

THE DELINEATOR.   NOVEMBER, 1901.

Victorians in winter hats. *The Delineator*, November 1901.

Many books were dedicated to beauty routines that instructed women on how to attack time and nature. Two full hours per day were recommended to carry out a proper beauty regimen. Women chose to endure their timely grooming practices so as not to appear plain and unattractive.

The toilette for men consisted of Eau de Cologne, hair pomade, and shaving soap. Dandies were still around in the early part of the century. They were easy targets for satirical illustrations that showed off their excessive use of cosmetics and fashion.

The Great Exhibition of 1851 held in Hyde Park, London, England, showcased rich displays of cosmetics, soaps, and fancy toiletries and created a high demand for items associated with grooming. Heliotrope and lilac were popular scents for toilette waters. The use of musk-based fragrances gained popularity by 1912.

The nineteenth century ushered in large-scale immigration to America and Australia from Europe. Many people brought household care handbooks. Included were recipes for the most popular preparations from their native lands, making it possible for settlers to enjoy the use of their favorite cosmetics.

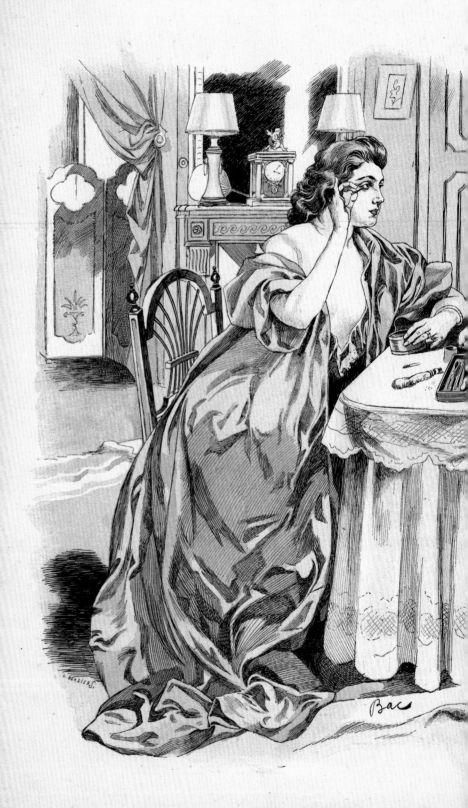

LES DAMES PASTELLISTES

— Il va hurler, mais tant pis.

Woman applies eye makeup. Illustration from *La Femme Intime*, 1894.

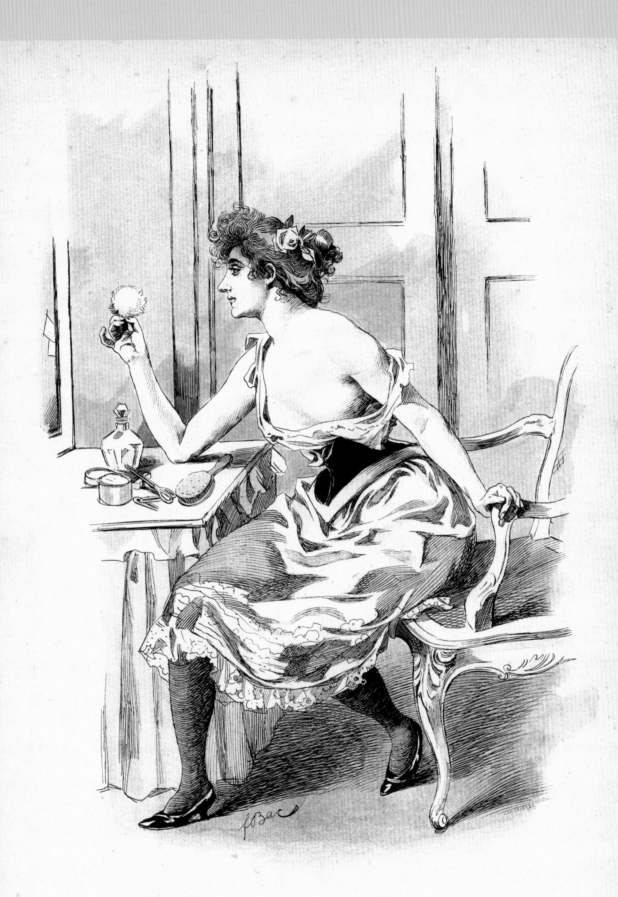

— Ils ne se doutent pas du mal qu'on se donne.

Woman at boudoir. Illustration from *La Femme Intime*, 1894.

In 1804, Napoleon Bonaparte crowned himself Emperor of France and lifted the restrictions of perfume production. Napoleon favored scented soap and cologne.

Empress Josephine, queen of France and Napoleon's first wife, favored a heavily rouged cheek. She spent large sums of money on her supply of rouge. Many women still purchased rouge under the counter from the local chemist shop.

Many cosmetic items of the time, especially liquid and cream rouge, contained metallic ingredients that were harmful to the skin. Some powders contained non-harmful rice starch or bismuth, but the minerals in these powders turned black when exposed to sulfur from the coal fires that burned throughout the home.

In the 1890s, bright red lip salves, similar to current lipsticks used today, were applied. Before then, lips were touched with face cream or rouge.

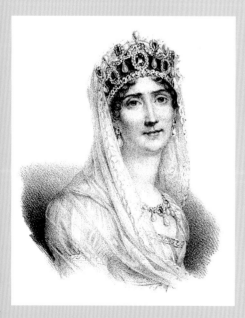

Portrait of Josephine, empress of France, 1830.

44

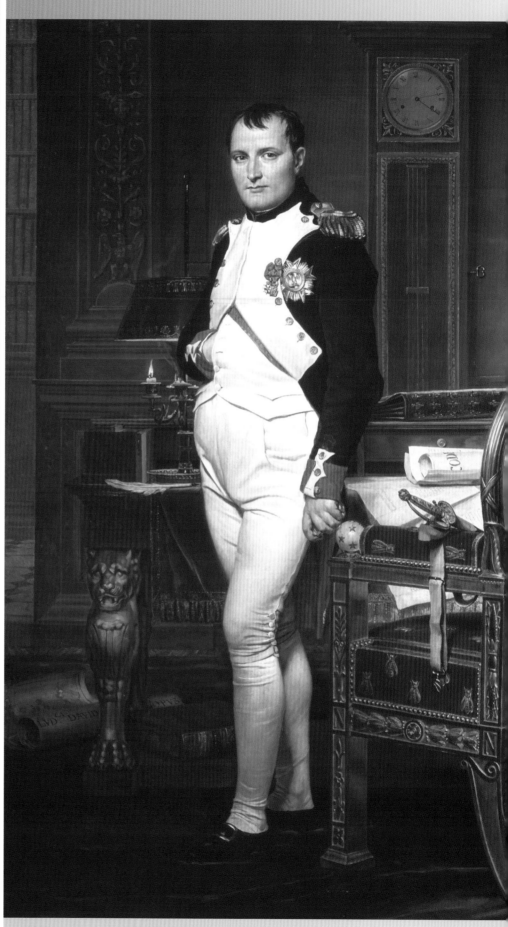

Portrait of Napoleon Bonaparte by Jacques-Louis David, 1812.

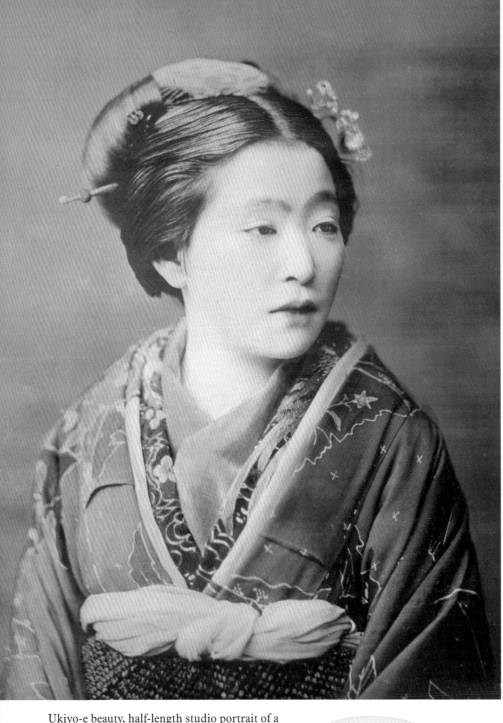

Ukiyo-e beauty, half-length studio portrait of a woman, facing slightly right. c. 1877.

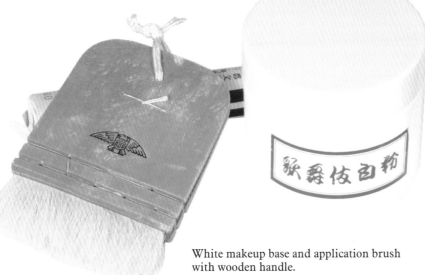

White makeup base and application brush with wooden handle.

Pomades for the hair and hands were in use throughout Europe. These perfumed fat concoctions tamed the hair and softened the hands at night. Gloves with ointments were worn to bed in order to keep the hands soft and smooth.

Trade with the Orient brought images of geishas, maharani, and other Asian beauties to Victorian women. They dressed in costumes for parties inspired by these exotic looks.

Toward the end of the nineteenth century, cosmetics were in abundance and affordable to most social classes. The use of cosmetics was an accepted and important practice for most women of the time. Cosmetics became a commercialized commodity complete with eye-catching packaging and clever advertising slogans. In 1886, Harriet Hubbard Ayer introduced her famous cream endorsed by celebrity Lillie Langtry. In the 1890s, Helena Rubinstein went to Australia with the recipe for her mother's skin cream.

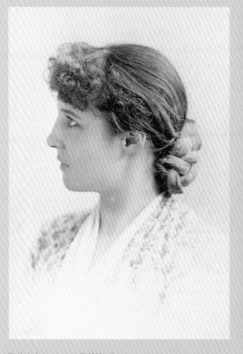

British actress Lillie Langtry, c. 1900.

45

Historical TIMELINE

A.D. 1900 to A.D. 1918

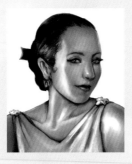

Helena Rubinstein opens her beauty shop and uses a relative's formulas for her cold cream, astringent, and vanishing cream.

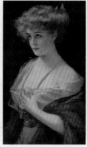

1903
Richard Hudnut manufactures the DuBarry line in the United States. The line is named after the Comtesse Jeanne DuBarry, known to exude "the essence of femininity."

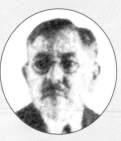

1905
The bosom is emphasized in fashions. Colored shadow is dusted on the cleavage and pale blue veins are painted on the chest to enhance the breasts.

1908
Max Factor opens his makeup studio in Los Angeles for the film industry. The studio makes wigs from real hair.

1900
The Edwardian beauty is voluptuous. She sports a rounded face and a white and pink complexion achieved by the heavy use of powder and rouge.

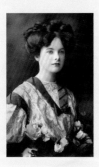

1902
Charles Dana Gibson draws the Gibson Girl, who represents the ideal woman of the time. The hair is waved and worn pinned-up. Skin is lightened with Blanc de Perles, a powder made with pearls. Dresses accentuate a narrow-waisted, hourglass silhouette.

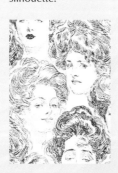

1904
Ruth Maurer creates the Marinello Company, which later establishes a franchise of beauty schools.

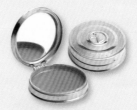

You owe it to yourself next time to get the
NEWEST AND MOST IMPROVED
MACHINELESS
PERMANENT
MARINELLO BEAUTY SHOP

1906
The Food and Drug Act prohibits cosmetics mislabeling and requires proof of claims.

1909
Newspapers advertise Pompeian skin cream.

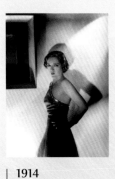

1914
World War I changes women's hairstyles from long to short since working in factories makes long hair impractical and dangerous. Mary Pickford became America's sweetheart as a tomboy urchin in silent films.

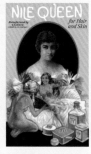

1918
A group of African American investors forms the Kashmir Chemical Co. and produces Nile Queen cosmetics, a brand of products aimed at the African American consumer.

1910
The Gillette Company advertises the safety razor and promotes self-shaving for men.

1915
Helena Rubinstein opens her salon on Fifth Avenue in New York City.

Only one in five Americans uses any kind of toiletry preparations.

T. L. Williams creates the Maybelline Company.

1916
Shalimar perfume is introduced. Its musky Oriental scent is popularized by the trend toward exotic looks and foreign fashions.

Dorothy Gray establishes her New York salon.

1912
A woman's handbag contains lipstick, an eyebrow pencil, a small flask of scent, and a gold or silver compact with pressed powder in shades of white, flesh, or Rachel.

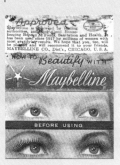

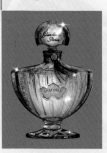

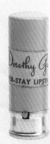

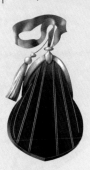

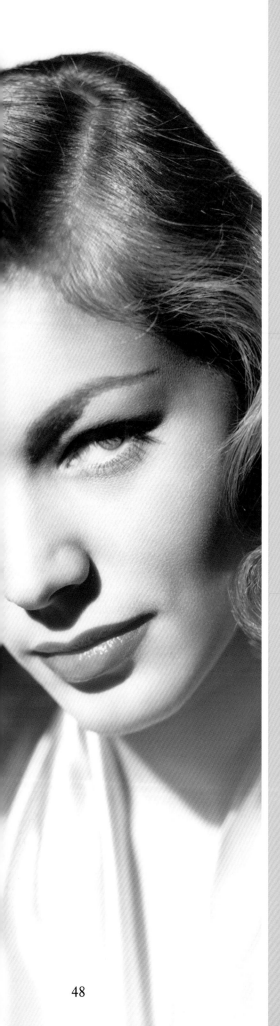

The Eyes

The eyes are not only the windows to the soul, but powerful communication tools. A simple glance can reveal the true intentions of its sender. Throughout time, makeup has played a prominent role in accentuating the eyes. Historical eras and time periods can be identified by observing the specific colors, trends, and styles used to decorate the eye.

Black pigments in the forms of kohl and mascara were used for centuries to darken lashes, eyelids, and eyebrows. The Egyptians had many options for eyebrow dyes. Very exotic mixtures involved crocodile earth and donkey's liver that were rolled into dye balls. Kohl was commonly made of malachite, galena copper, iron manganese, and lead. These minerals were ground up with a stone slab and kept in shells or small alabaster containers. Kohl was mixed with oil or fat and applied with a shaped stick. Lampblack was an inexpensive eye paint concocted by burning a candle and collecting the black soot left from the flame.

During the 1800s, the use of eyelash and eyebrow darkeners was acceptable for those born with fair hair, which was viewed as a birth defect. Such people were instructed to cook up a hair dye made with walnut hulls to darken the hair to a light brown.

1910 saw a shift from home production of cosmetics to commercially manufactured production. A 1909 performance of the London Ballet featured the use of heavy eye shadows and mascara, and spurred the brisk sale of these products. The upper classes favored kohl on the eyes, and eye shadow colors were coordinated to match clothing. Gold and silver eye shadows were also introduced to use with eveningwear.

After seeing Russian dancers use heavier eye makeup on stage, Elizabeth Arden and Helena Rubinstein were inspired to create bold eye makeup for their upscale customers. Helena Rubinstein wrote in her autobiography, "I experimented privately and learned many valuable lessons from stage personalities, which in turn I taught to a few of my more daring clients. They spread the word, and I knew that another beauty barrier would soon be toppled." Through her relationships with fashion influencers such as the Russian dancers, she was able to break down years of taboos associated with eye cosmetics.

The smoky gaze of Lauren Bacall, the 1940s screen siren Humphrey Bogart called "Baby," was legendary.

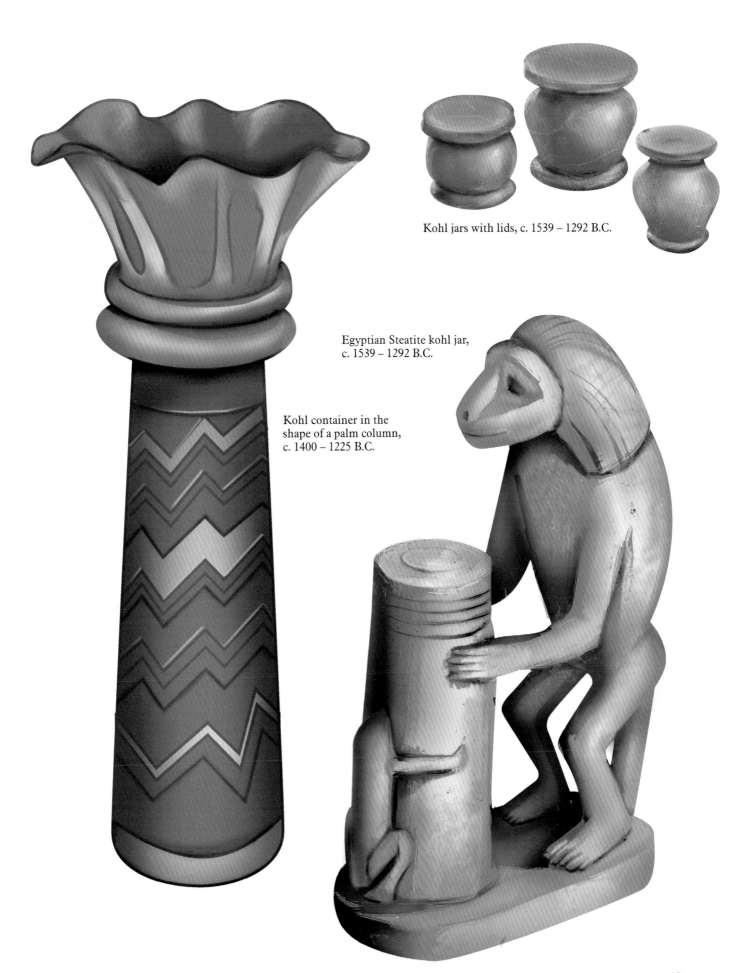

Kohl jars with lids, c. 1539 – 1292 B.C.

Egyptian Steatite kohl jar,
c. 1539 – 1292 B.C.

Kohl container in the
shape of a palm column,
c. 1400 – 1225 B.C.

By the end of World War I, the hair dye for men called mascaro was converted into the word mascara and re-sold with a new purpose: to beautify and darken lashes.

In 1926, Rudolph Valentino starred in the silent movie *The Son of the Sheik*, setting off a wave of Egyptian revivalism and Orientalism in American popular culture.

Screen actresses played a major role in the spread of mascara use. Their expressive eyes were all they had to convey emotion on the silent screen. The use of mascara to lengthen the lashes was a way for the important eyes to take center stage in camera close-ups.

Theda Bara was the first to adopt the heavily kohled eyes developed by Helena Rubinstein. Her dark rimmed eyes became her trademark, which she wore on-screen and off. The look was so revolutionary, it was reported on by every major newspaper.

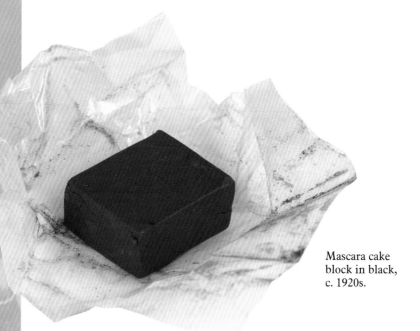

Mascara cake block in black, c. 1920s.

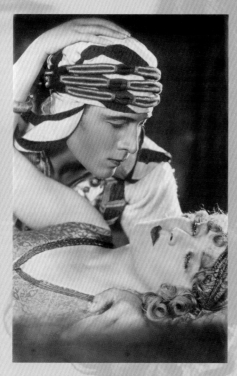

Rudolph Valentino and Vilma Banky in *The Son of The Sheik*, 1926.

50

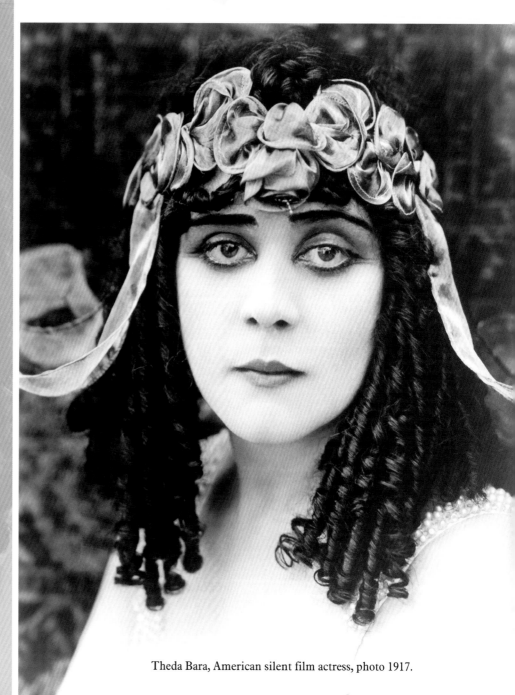

Theda Bara, American silent film actress, photo 1917.

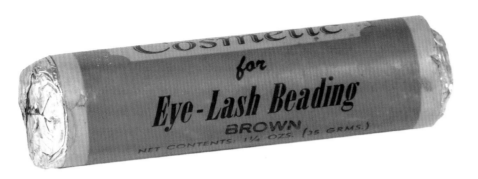

Cosmetic Eye-Lash Beading wax in brown, c. 1920s.

During the 1920s, Max Factor invented his own version of mascara called Cosmetique. His formula, specifically developed for Hollywood actress Clara Bow, was a waxy substance that came wrapped in a thin foil roll, which resembled a thick crayon. This concoction was used by slicing off a piece and melting it over a flame, then dipping an orange stick in the hot wax and applying it in an upward motion on the lashes. The wax thickened the lashes, but made the hair stick together, especially with changes in the temperature of the wax under the hot studio lights. Removal of the wax was taken care of with heavy cold cream.

Max Factor's Supreme Eyelash and Eyebrow Masque, c. 1928.

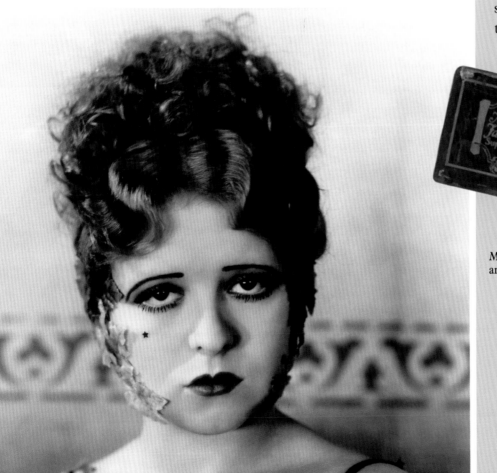

Clara Bow, Hollywood screen starlet, photo c. 1920s.

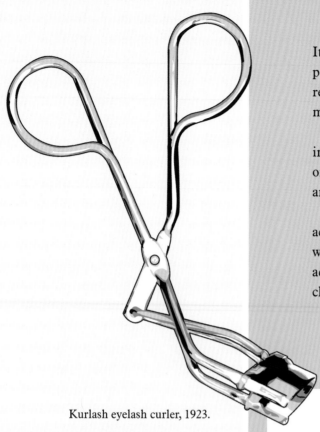

Kurlash, a type of eyelash curling device, was invented in 1923. It was costly and very time consuming to use. It took ten minutes per eye for results. As the first device of its kind, it gained praise and recognition because it worked to give the lashes curl and make them more prominent on the face.

The eyebrow pencil of the 1920s rose to popularity after it was improved with a new formula consisting of hydrogenated cottonseed oil. This new ingredient made the texture and its application softer and also prevented the spread of harmful bacteria.

The eyebrow pencil and mascara were favorite items of many actresses. Greta Garbo's pale blond lashes and eyebrows were defined with applications of mascara and eye pencils. Her look was greatly admired and copied by women. She was recognized as the ultimate classic face of beauty.

Kurlash eyelash curler, 1923.

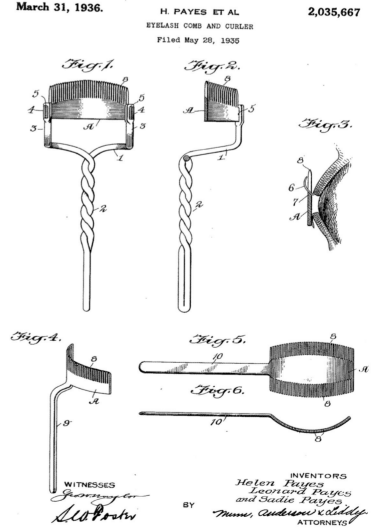

Eyelash Comb and Curler patent, no. 2,035,667. H. Payes, 1935.

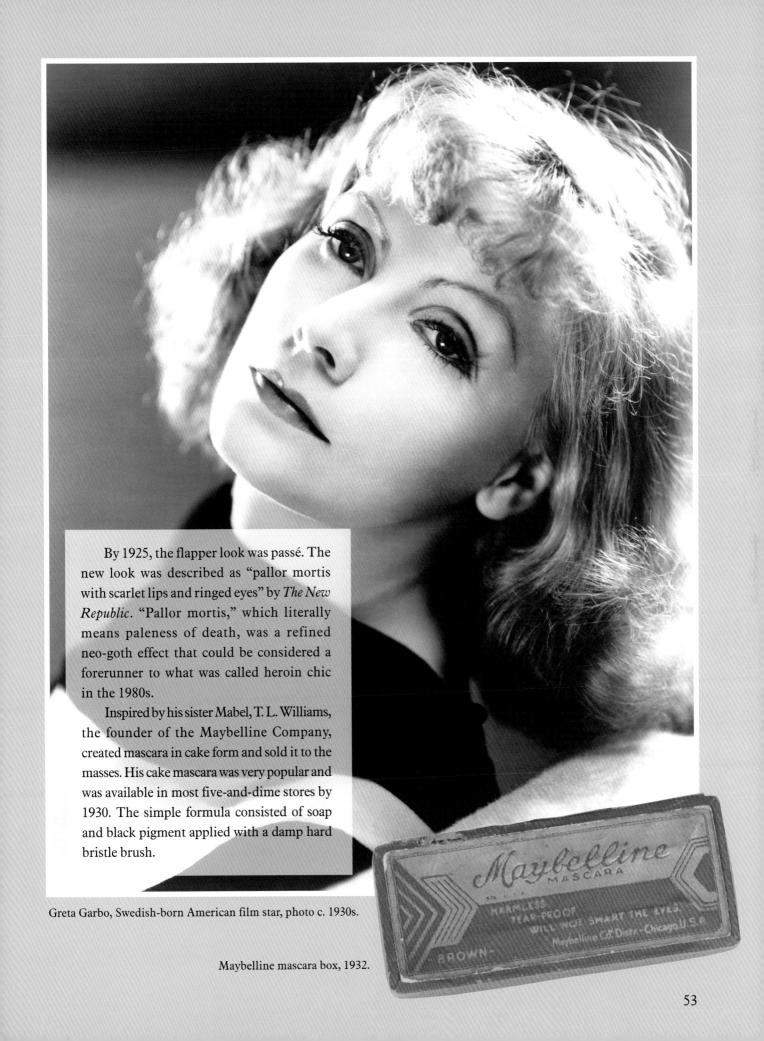

By 1925, the flapper look was passé. The new look was described as "pallor mortis with scarlet lips and ringed eyes" by *The New Republic*. "Pallor mortis," which literally means paleness of death, was a refined neo-goth effect that could be considered a forerunner to what was called heroin chic in the 1980s.

Inspired by his sister Mabel, T. L. Williams, the founder of the Maybelline Company, created mascara in cake form and sold it to the masses. His cake mascara was very popular and was available in most five-and-dime stores by 1930. The simple formula consisted of soap and black pigment applied with a damp hard bristle brush.

Greta Garbo, Swedish-born American film star, photo c. 1930s.

Maybelline mascara box, 1932.

By 1936, sixty-two percent of women used mascara regularly. Even the depression years did not suppress the appetite for cosmetic use. Cheap novelty products flooded the market and allowed thrifty women to spend their spare change. Cosmetics were considered essentials to women seeking employment outside the home.

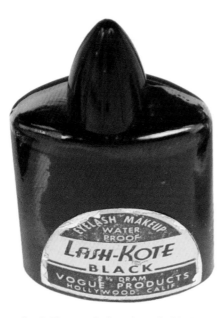

Lash-Kote eyelash makeup in black, c. 1950s.

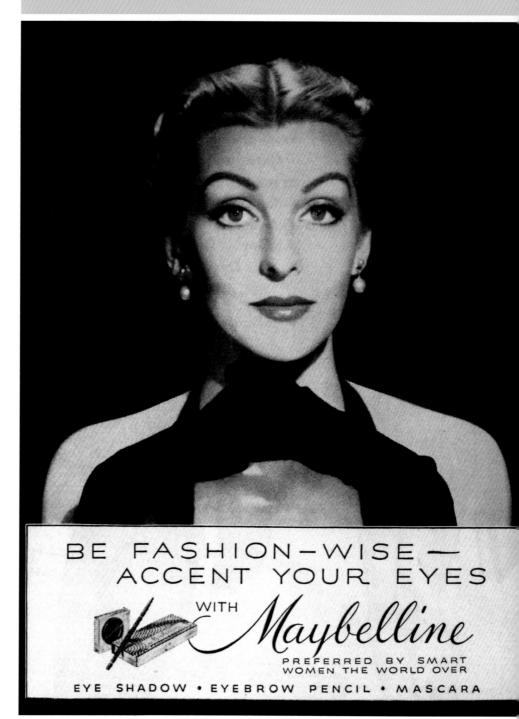

BE FASHION-WISE—
ACCENT YOUR EYES
WITH *Maybelline*
PREFERRED BY SMART
WOMEN THE WORLD OVER
EYE SHADOW • EYEBROW PENCIL • MASCARA

Maybelline eye cosmetics advertisement, 1952.

Maybelline mascara box, 1939.

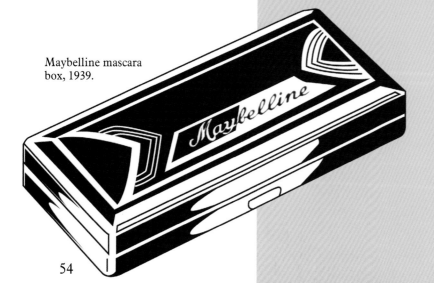

Cream mascara was introduced in the late 1920s. It consisted of dyed Vaseline and was applied by squeezing a small amount from the tube to the brush. Two popular brands were Tattoo and Laleek Longlash.

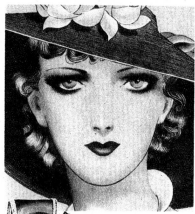

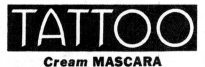
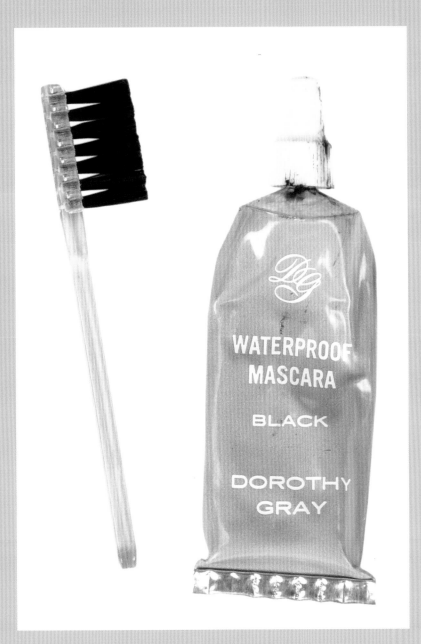

Dorothy Gray Waterproof Mascara in black, c. 1940.

Tattoo Cream Mascara advertisement, c. 1940s.

Liquid mascaras did not become popular until 1958 with Helena Rubinstein's MascaraMatic. The container resembled a long pen with a grooved metal tip at the end that held the product for application.

The patent that most resembled the modern mascara bottle was granted to Frank L. Engel Jr. in 1939 for his shoe blackening bottle mechanism. Unfortunately, Mr. Engel did not profit from his patent. The idea for mascara wands did not take off until the late 1950s after his claim expired.

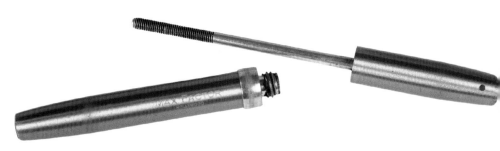

Max Factor mascara, hairless wand in brown/black, in gold metal tube, 1958.

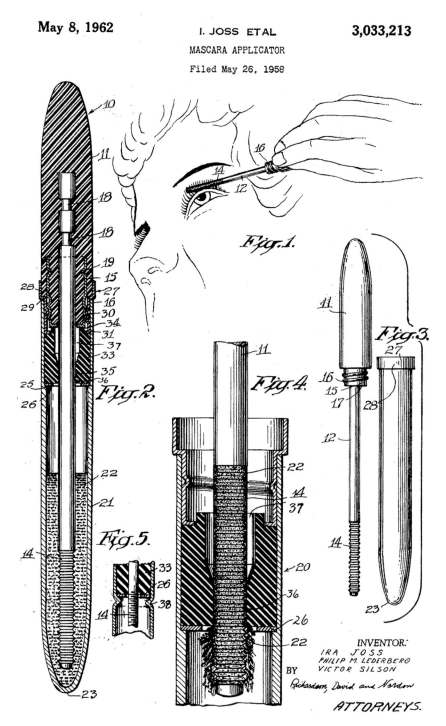

Mascara Applicator patent, no. 3,033,213. I. Joss, 1958.

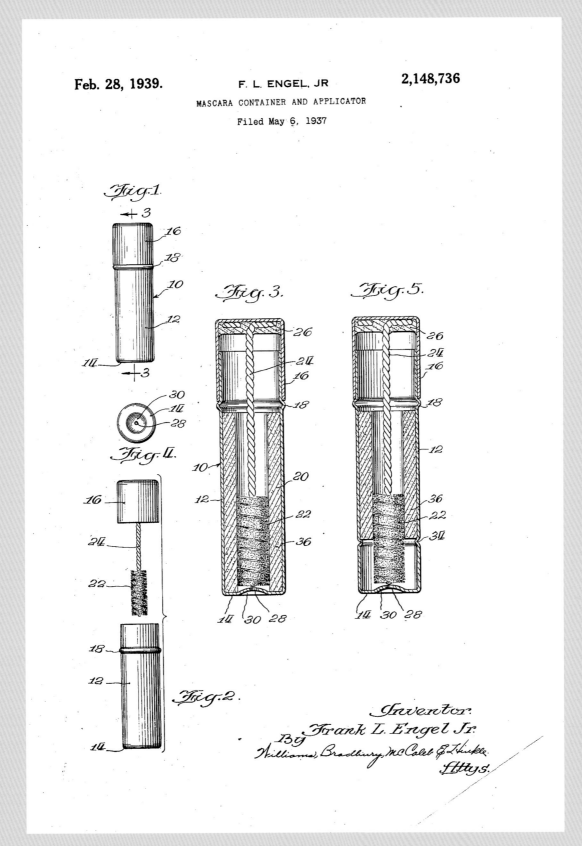

Mascara Container and Applicator patent, no. 2,148,736. F. L. Engel Jr., 1937.

Many other advances followed the introduction of the MascaraMatic, ushering the development of the current mascara wand. New materials found by breaking down petroleum products brought better formulas for mascara. New solvents improved the drying time that led to the creation of products like liquid eyeliners. In the 1950s, Audrey Hepburn's doe-eyes encouraged women to experiment with looks more than ever.

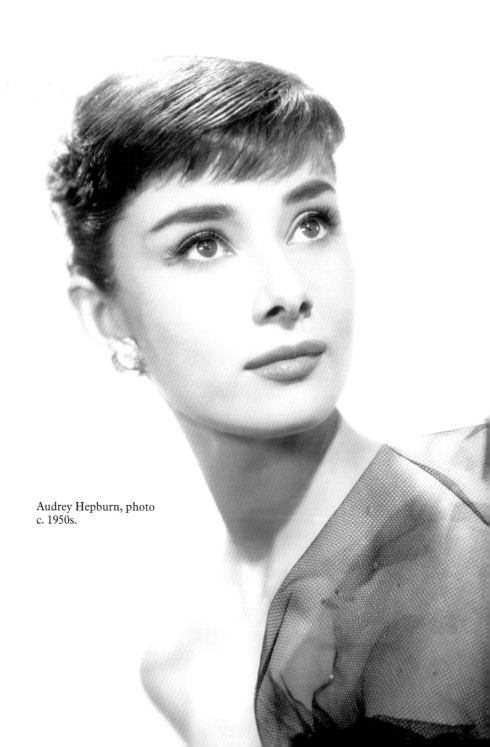

Audrey Hepburn, photo
c. 1950s.

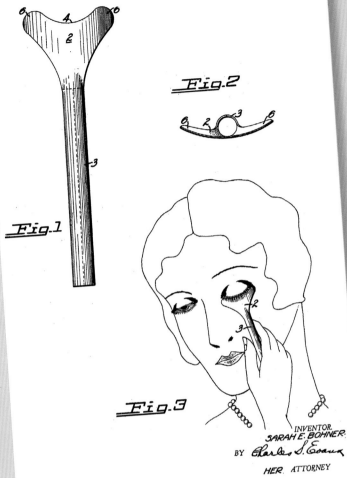

Aug. 23, 1932.

S. E. BOHNER

EYELID GUARD

Filed Oct. 20, 1931

1,873,928

Fig.2

Fig.1

Fig.3

INVENTOR.
SARAH E. BOHNER.

BY _Charles S. Evans_

HER ATTORNEY

Eyelid Guard patent, no.
1,873,928. S. E. Bohner, 1931.

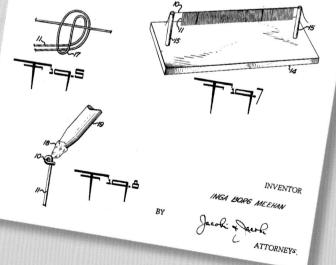

May 1, 1962

Filed Jan. 13, 1959

I. B. MEEHAN
ARTIFICIAL EYELASHES AND METHOD
AND APPARATUS FOR MAKING SAME

3,032,042

2 Sheets—Sheet 1

INVENTOR
INGA BORG MEEHAN

BY

Jacobi + Jacobi

ATTORNEYS.

Artificial Eyelashes and Method and
Apparatus for Making Same patent,
no. 3,032,042. I. B. Meehan, 1962.

In 1971, Maybelline's Great Lash water-based mascara was introduced to the market. With its distinctive green and pink tube, it is still the number-one selling mascara in the marketplace.

The first colorless mascara was introduced in 1988 by the Max Factor company. This product was instrumental in achieving the popular "no makeup" look.

From the 1990s through the first decade of the new millennium and beyond, mascara has become much more sophisticated in terms of function. Mascara formulas for eyelashes have been created to add volume, lengthen, curl, and even to promote eyelash growth.

Researchers have developed bold, vivid pigments evolving into a myriad of colors in mascara and eye liner products. Waterproof, metallic, and bright colors have given consumers a vast number of choices when looking for color around the eye.

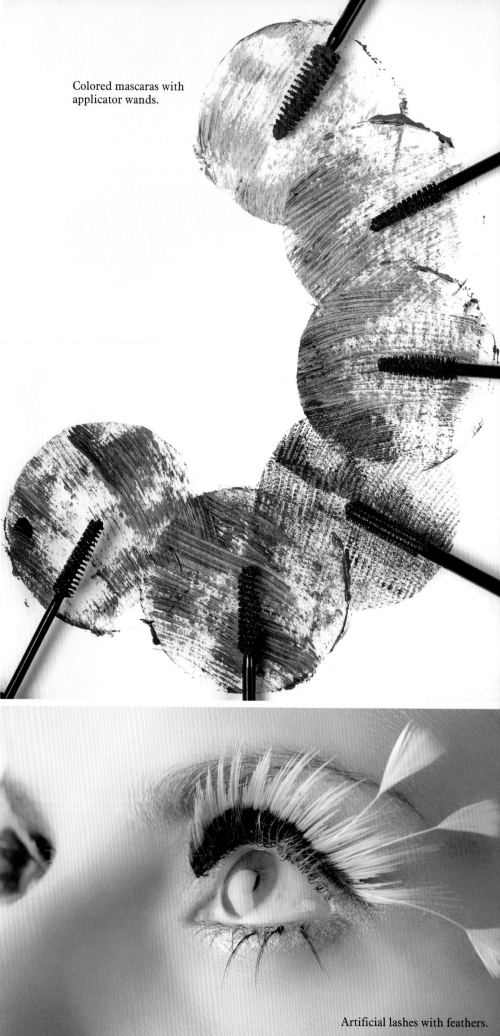

Colored mascaras with applicator wands.

Artificial lashes with feathers.

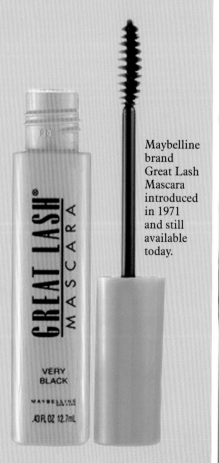

Maybelline brand Great Lash Mascara introduced in 1971 and still available today.

GREAT LASH MASCARA

VERY BLACK

MAYBELLINE

.43 FL OZ 12.7mL

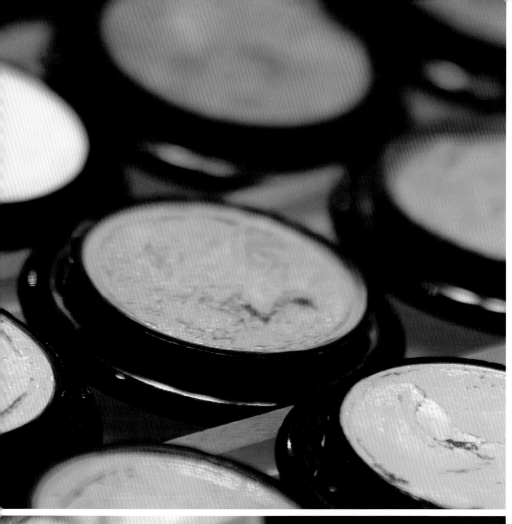

New designs in false lashes that used bright colors, feathers, or crystals introduced fantasy to the eye. These were made popular by celebrities like Madonna and Christina Aguilera.

Gel eye liners and cream-based shadows that did not smear or flake provided an alternative to pencils and liquids that did so. Colors available ranged from neutrals to striking neons. These formulas boasted additional benefits like de-puffing compounds and no-budge, all-day performance.

Cream-based eye shadows.

Cosmetic powders for eyes.

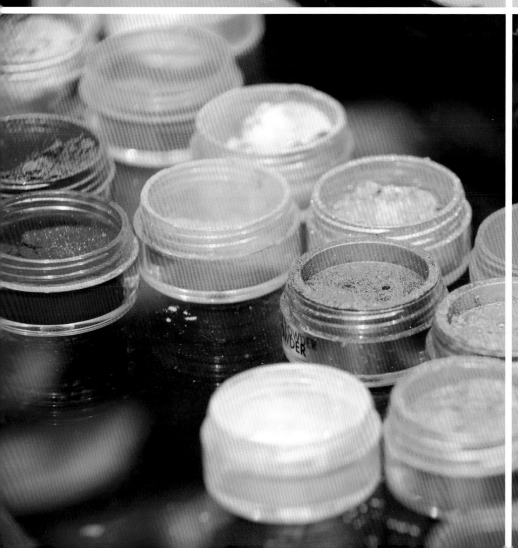

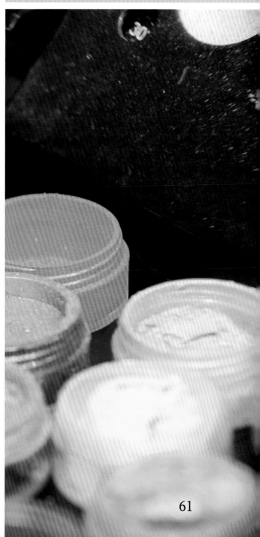

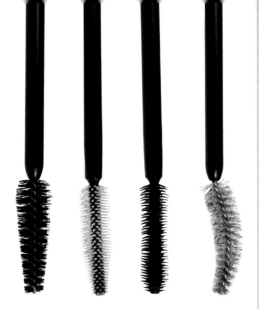

Mascara applicator wands.

New technology in brush manufacturing led to silicone-molded brushes that held more product and produced a thicker mascara application. The "fat lash" was achieved with a combination of larger, thicker brushes and creamy, buildable formulas. Mascaras contained vitamins and hair strengthening compounds to keep lashes healthy as well as made-up.

Estée Lauder's
new
Automatic Creme Eyeshadow

It smooths on like a creme, dries like a powder and has the soft shimmer of pure silk.

Automatic is the key word. Every time you pull out the spongetip applicator, you get precisely the right amount of velvet creme shadow that smooths on perfectly, blends softly and dries in a moment to a crease-proof, smudge-proof, waterproof finish. A silken finish that holds its own all day long. There is simply nothing else you could want in an eyeshadow. And it took Estée Lauder and today's technology to bring it to you.

Estée Lauder

Eight soft, silken shades:
Blue Haze   Misty Turquoise   Polished Pewter   Fresh Water Green
Hickory Brown   Dusk Blue   Smoky Iris   Crystal Peach Highlighter

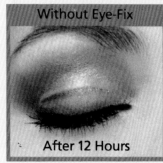

Estée Lauder brand Automatic Creme Eyeshadow advertisement, 1976.

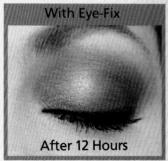

the breakthrough way beautiful all day, all night.

ONLY EYE-FIX HAS PRIMILIN III.
IT WORKS—TESTS PROVE IT.

Without Eye-Fix	With Eye-Fix
After 12 Hours	After 12 Hours

Eyelids are unretouched.

CONTROLS CREASING, STREAKING, FADING.
- Eyeshadow glides on like silk, blends perfectly.
- Keeps eye makeup color-true, perfect all day, all night.

ADDS PRECIOUS MOISTURE.
- Brings vital moisture to the delicate eye area which is so prone to aging.
- With continued use, provides long-term moisturization benefits.

FEELS SO SHEER AND LIGHT.
- Invisible. You can't see it or feel it when it's on.
- Colorless. Contains no frost or tint to distort eyeshadow color.

Eye-Fix is specially formulated and tested for the delicate eye area.

Elizabeth Arden

DERMATOLOGIST, CLINICALLY, ALLERGY TESTED. FRAGRANCE FREE.

A booklet with documented proof is available at the Elizabeth Arden counter.

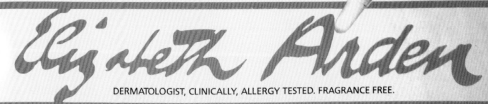

Elizabeth Arden brand Eye Fix Primer advertisement, 1984.

Formulas have become lighter and loaded with beneficial ingredients. New elastic polymer formulas have created mascaras to thicken and stretch lashes beyond their normal length. Others have added silk fibers to make lashes appear thicker. Enriched with natural oils, some formulas have delivered a glossy black finish, while others dried quickly for a matted smoke-black look.

The future of eye makeup has brought a closer fusion of fashion with science, giving consumers beautiful colors while promoting healthy eyes and lashes.

"I don't believe my eyes!"

Introducing new 'Shiny Shadows', the gleamiest shadows ever! Just slick 'em on with your fingertip, and your eyes simply light up with shine. The secret: Cleanshine. Shine that goes on creamy, stays on clean. In shades that are soft and shimmery, polished and pretty. Try new 'Shiny Shadows'. For the clean, natural look of Cover Girl Eyes!

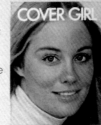

COVER GIRL

Cover Girl and actress Cybill Shepherd

New Shiny Shadows™ From Cover Girl Eyes®

CoverGirl brand Shiny Shadows advertisement, model Cybill Shepherd, 1973.

Helena Rubinstein eye cosmetics for Univis brand eyewear, 1976.

Aziza brand eye cosmetics advertisement, 1986.

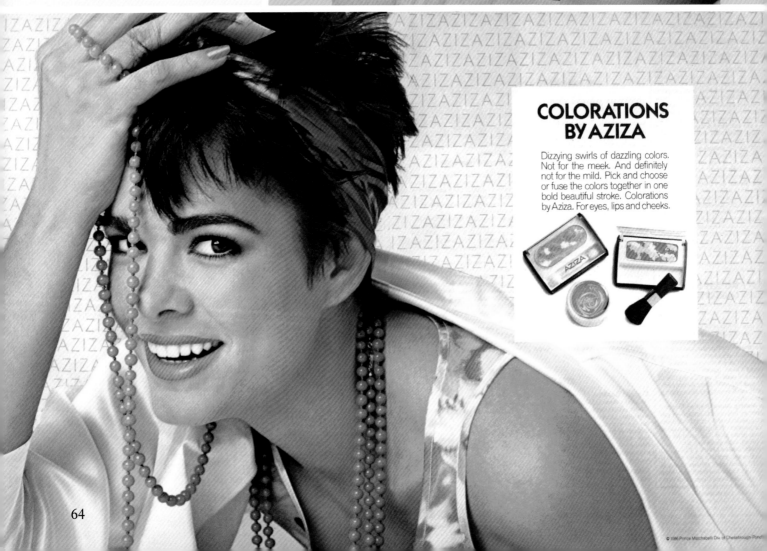

Announcing the end of the conflict between your eyewear and your eye makeup.

HELENA RUBINSTEIN AND UNIVIS INTRODUCE THE FIRST COORDINATED LOOK

EYE MYSTIQUE At last. Helena Rubinstein and Univis have created a special new look in eye allure.
Eye Mystique.
A collection of eight great new fashion frames by Univis in 14 subtly scintillating colors coordinated to eye makeup by Helena Rubinstein.
Eye Mystique.
With coordinated colors that work with your eye makeup, not against it, to give you a more flattering look. And unlike some frames that dominate your face, Eye Mystique frames

are so soft, so naturally sculptured, they enhance the contours of your own face.
Now you can't go wrong. No matter what your individual style, Eye Mystique has a wide range of unique colors and designs coordinated to add new dazzle and excitement to your most attractive feature.
Your professional eyecare or eyewear specialist has the Eye Mystique frame collection ready to show you, along with a Helena Rubinstein Guide to Beautiful Eyes to help you achieve your own coordinated look.

UNIVIS
Itek Ophthalmic Products

COLORATIONS BY AZIZA

Dizzying swirls of dazzling colors. Not for the meek. And definitely not for the mild. Pick and choose or fuse the colors together in one bold beautiful stroke. Colorations by Aziza. For eyes, lips and cheeks.

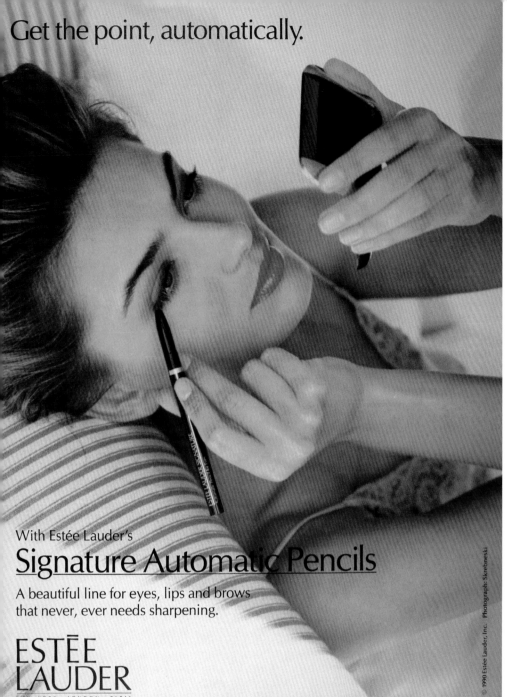

Get the point, automatically.

With Estée Lauder's

Signature Automatic Pencils

A beautiful line for eyes, lips and brows
that never, ever needs sharpening.

ESTĒE LAUDER
NEW YORK · LONDON · PARIS

© 1990 Estée Lauder, Inc.   Photograph: Skrebneski

Estée Lauder brand Signature Automatic Pencils advertisement, 1990.

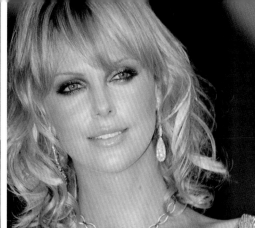

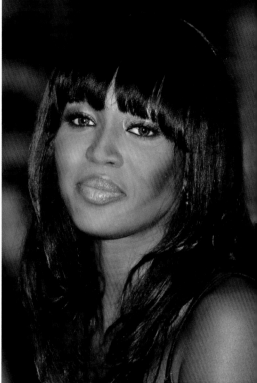

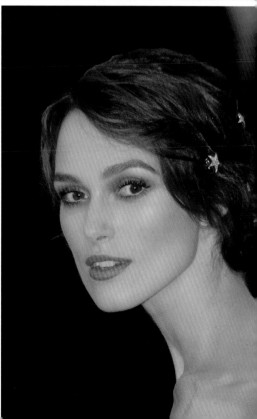

Top:
Charlize Theron, international film star, photo 2003.

Middle:
Naomi Campbell, British supermodel, photo 2008.

Bottom:
Keira Knightley, British actress, photo 2007.

The Lips

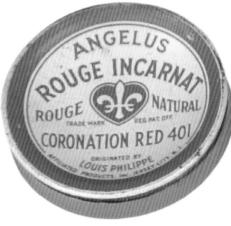

Angelus Rouge Incarnat in Coronation Red, 1935.

Lip colors are considered the most widely used cosmetics ever invented. Women who typically do not wear a full face of makeup commonly wear lipstick. From the earliest of civilizations to present time, women throughout history have painted their lips. The Hindus used betel to darken the lips and teeth, and the Elizabethans painted the lips with a colored plaster pencil. Lipstick formulas included items such as dried and crushed insect bodies, cochineal, beeswax, and olive oil.

Rouge was used both as a lip colorant and as a cheek paint. Because of its popularity and use of easily found ingredients, many recipes to prepare rouge creams or powders existed. Until the Revolution in America when patriots left behind the customs of the English aristocracy, men also wore rouge. One of the first to manufacture rouge in the United States was Samson American in 1860, who crafted rouge from alkanet, oil of turpentine, and oil of roses. It was advertised as giving the cheeks a look of perfect health. In 1867, Harriet Fish patented a rouge pad to use on the cheeks and lips. The formula was created from carmine, beets, strawberries, and hollyhock root.

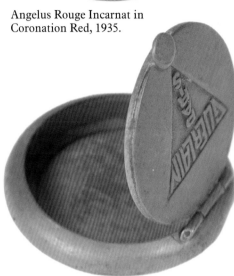

Guerlain rouge, c. 1840.

Around 1880, the Guerlain Company produced one of the first commercially successful lipstick products. This lipstick pomade was formulated from grapefruit mixed with butter and wax. Other vendors tried to compete with their inferior products, which contained ingredients that irritated the skin and created thick and unnatural looking lips.

By World War I, chemical advances brought about synthetic reds that rendered a less dense, more natural appearance to the lips. With these new paints, lip color became socially acceptable and its usage was practiced freely across the country. Women were able to match the color of their lips to the outfits they wore, creating a market for many new colors of lipstick.

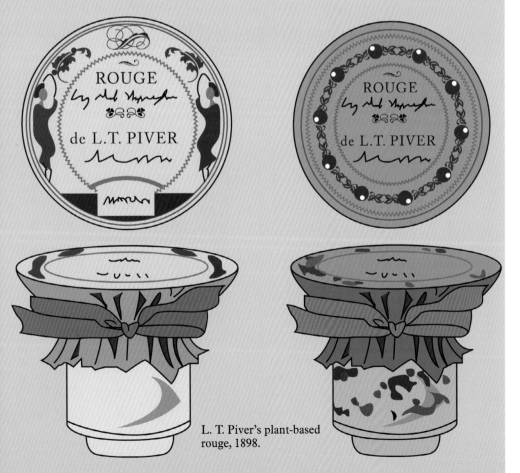

L. T. Piver's plant-based rouge, 1898.

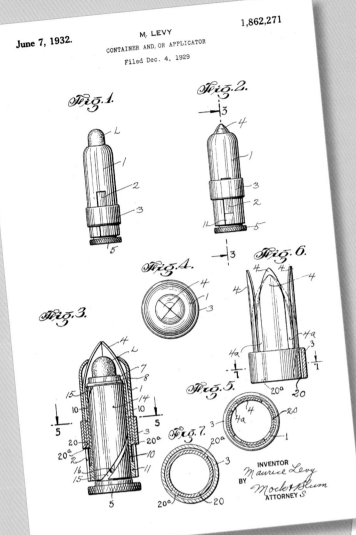

June 7, 1932.   M. LEVY   1,862,271
                        CONTAINER AND, OR APPLICATOR
                            Filed Dec. 4, 1929

In 1915, Maurice Levy designed the first American lipstick in a sliding metal tube. Before then, lip colors were sold in pots, on tinted papers, or in paper tubes. The first lipstick containers to swivel from the case were patented by James Bruce Mason Jr. in 1923. Named the Mason tube, the lipstick had a decorated screw at the bottom of the case that was turned to dispense product.

Container and, or Applicator patent, no. 1,862,271. M. Levy, 1929.

Dec. 28 , 1926.
                        G. W. NELSON   1,611,937
                          LIP STICK HOLDER
                          Filed May 25. 1926

Lip Stick Holder patent, no. 1,611,937. G. W. Nelson, 1926.

By 1924, it was estimated that 50 million American women used lipstick. During the 1920s, a tube of lipstick cost a dime. The use of cosmetics had transcended class structure because it was no longer confined to the wealthy or to usage on the stage. Women experimented with lip colors and shapes.

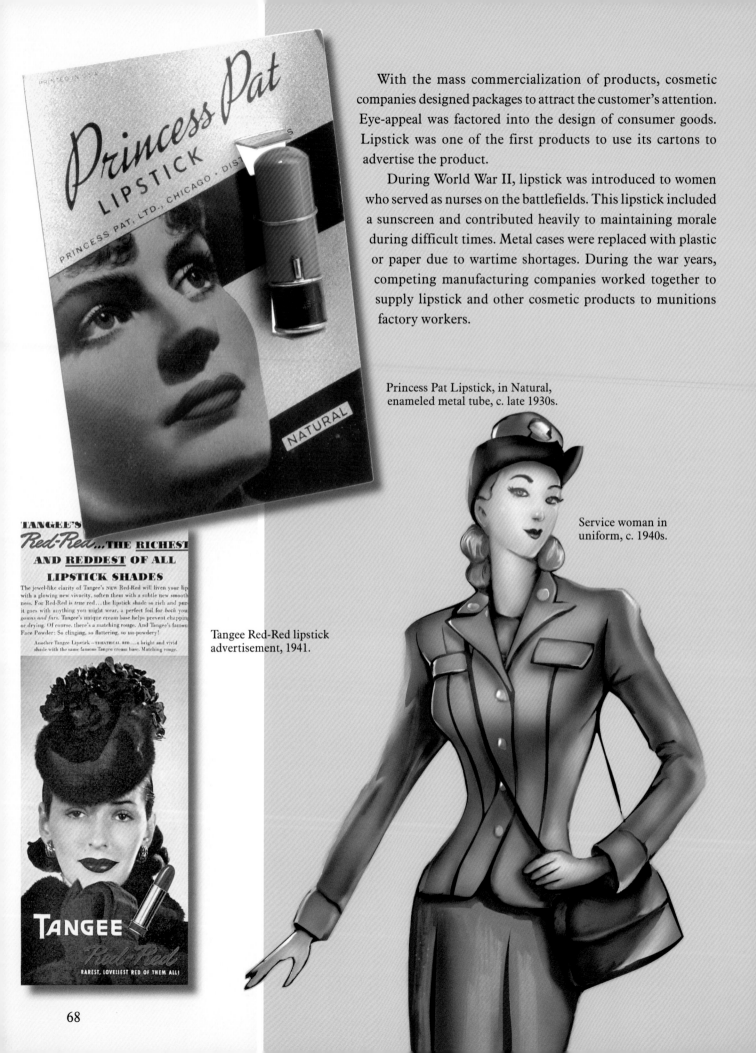

With the mass commercialization of products, cosmetic companies designed packages to attract the customer's attention. Eye-appeal was factored into the design of consumer goods. Lipstick was one of the first products to use its cartons to advertise the product.

During World War II, lipstick was introduced to women who served as nurses on the battlefields. This lipstick included a sunscreen and contributed heavily to maintaining morale during difficult times. Metal cases were replaced with plastic or paper due to wartime shortages. During the war years, competing manufacturing companies worked together to supply lipstick and other cosmetic products to munitions factory workers.

Princess Pat Lipstick, in Natural, enameled metal tube, c. late 1930s.

Service woman in uniform, c. 1940s.

Tangee Red-Red lipstick advertisement, 1941.

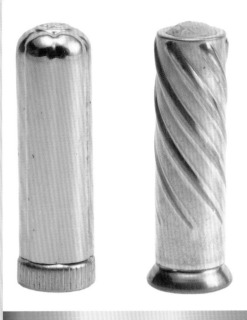

With their wide range of makeup products, Perc Westmore and Max Factor were pioneers who brought the magic of Hollywood to the average girl. These men were also responsible for creating the signature looks for the era's well known facial feature trends such as Clara Bow's cupid's bow lips and Joan Crawford's full lips.

Tangee lipstick was one of the first brands to target the younger consumer with a lipstick that changed color to suit the wearer. The lipstick provided a natural soft red color different from the opaque lip colors available at the time. Tangee became an acceptable transitional product as a girl blossomed into womanhood.

Hazel Bishop introduced the first no-smear lipstick in 1950. The formula was not "kiss proof" as was advertised, but it did present a change in the lipstick market as it spurred competition and more innovation in cosmetic formulas.

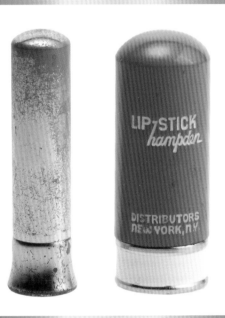

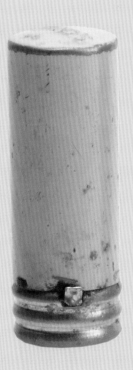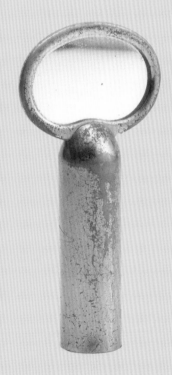

Pond's mini lipstick, made in England, c. late 1930s.

Mirrored brass lipstick topper, c. 1930.

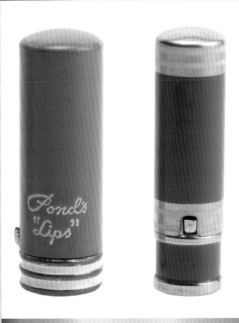

Top row, left to right:
Bourjois Evening in Paris lipstick in Ruby, brass metal tube, c. 1930.

Yardley lipstick in Natural Rose, brass top with plastic flower insert, c. late 1930s.

Middle row, left to right:
Lucien Lelong lipstick in Persuasion Rose, brass tube with swivel mechanism, c. late 1930s.

Hampden Lip-Stick in Ruby Red, enameled metal tube, c. late 1930s.

Bottom row, left to right:
Pond's "Lips" mini lipstick, enameled metal tube, c. 1930.

Ross Company Winx lipstick, enameled nickel tube, c. late 1930s.

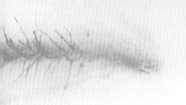

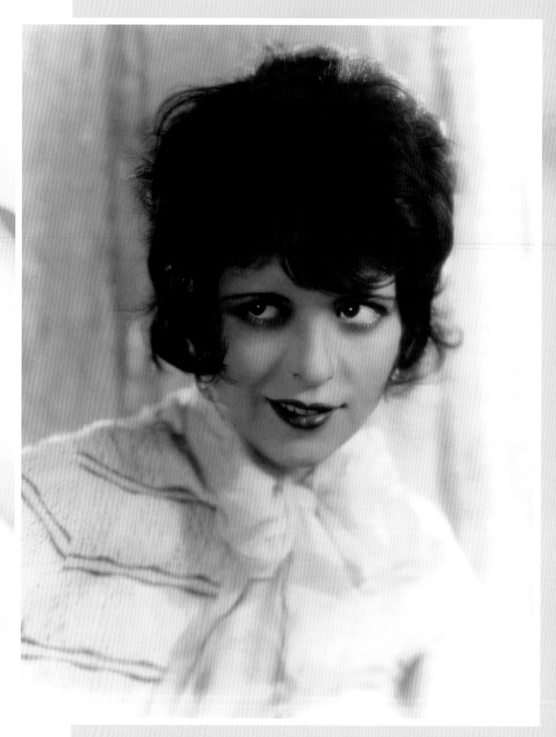

Clara Bow, photo, c. 1920s.

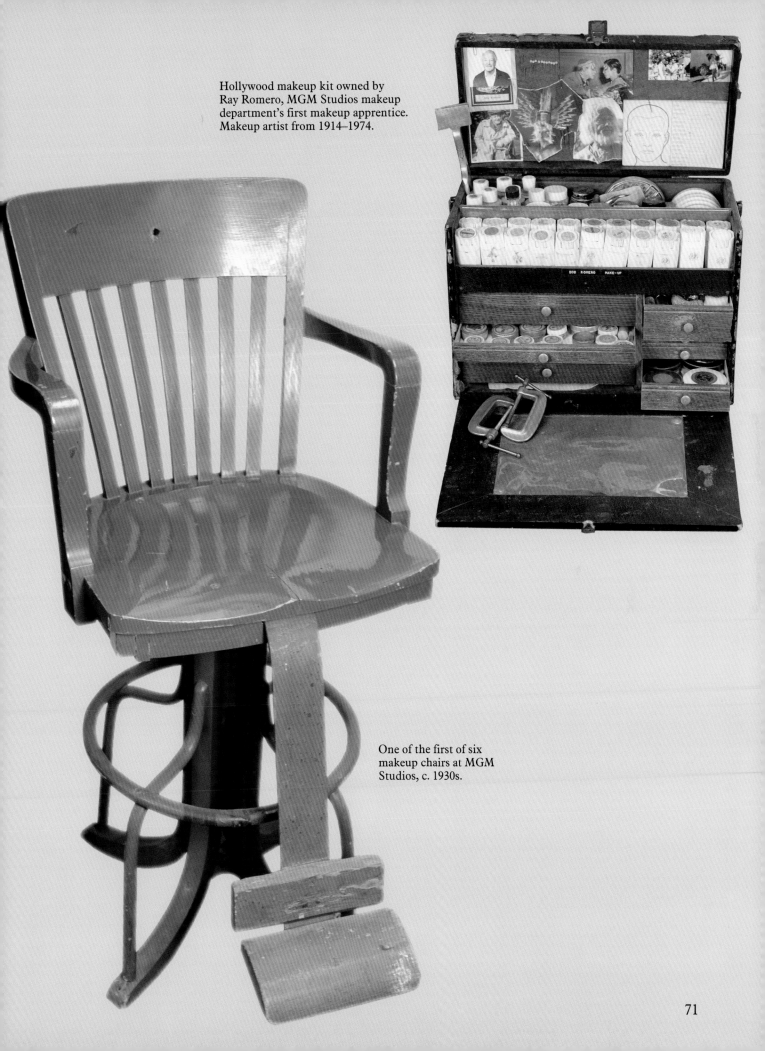

Hollywood makeup kit owned by
Ray Romero, MGM Studios makeup
department's first makeup apprentice.
Makeup artist from 1914–1974.

One of the first of six
makeup chairs at MGM
Studios, c. 1930s.

71

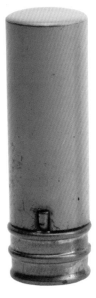

Woodbury brand lipstick in Raspberry, metal tube with enameled top, c. 1940s.

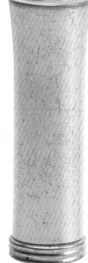

Irresistible brand lipstick in Persian Coral, brass tube, c. late 1940s.

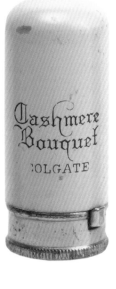

Colgate Company Cashmere Bouquet lipstick, enameled metal case, c. early 1940s.

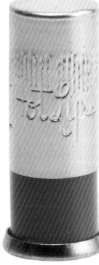
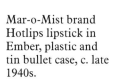

Mar-o-Mist brand Hotlips lipstick in Ember, plastic and tin bullet case, c. late 1940s.

From about the 1920s to the 1990s, lipstick technology focused on developing indelible long-lasting formulations, new colors, and new methods of packaging and applying lipstick. Early lipstick formulations were not highly durable. The color wax sticks of the past have been turned into a variety of textures with a multitude of uses. Multi-purpose colors were used on the lips and cheeks with new softer formulas. Lipstick was combined with gloss for a sheer and shiny finish and a lighter texture. Stains provided a natural flushed look to the lips applied with marker type applicators.

During the 1980s and '90s, manufacturers added mint to freshen breath with every lipstick application. Some of the innovations introduced to the lip category included moisture release colors, matte finishes for longer lasting color, sheer colors with moisture benefits, and colors with SPF (sun protection factor).

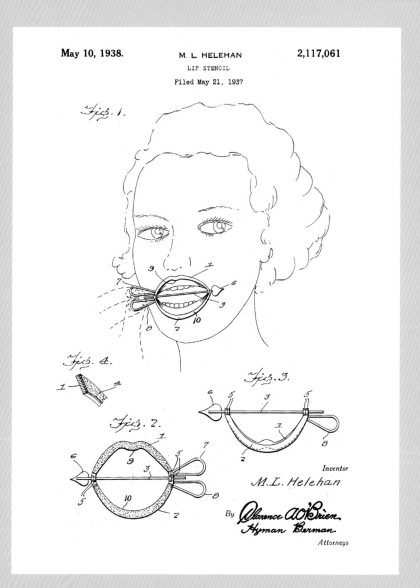

Lip Stencil patent, no. 2,117,061. M. L. Helehan, 1937.

Avon cosmetics brand Blossom Colors iridescent lipstick advertisement, c. 1960.

CoverGirl brand Medicated Lipstick by Noxzema advertisement, 1964.

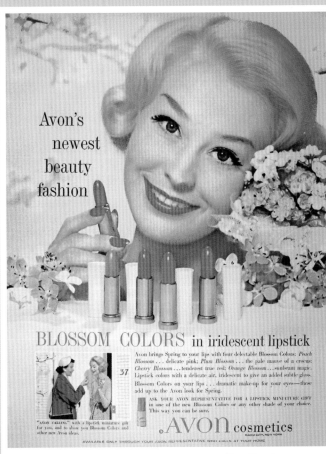

Avon's newest beauty fashion

BLOSSOM COLORS in iridescent lipstick

Avon brings Spring to your lips with four delectable Blossom Colors: *Peach Blossom* . . . delicate pink; *Plum Blossom* . . . the pale mauve of a crocus; *Cherry Blossom* . . . tenderest true red; *Orange Blossom* . . . sunbeam magic. Lipstick colors with a delicate air, iridescent to give an added subtle gloss. Blossom Colors on your lips . . . dramatic make-up for your eyes—these add up to the Avon look for Spring.

ASK YOUR AVON REPRESENTATIVE FOR A LIPSTICK MINIATURE GIFT in one of the new Blossom Colors or any other shade of your choice. This way you can be sure.

"AVON CALLING," with a lipstick miniature gift for you, and to show you Blossom Colors and other new Avon ideas.

AVON cosmetics
RADIO CITY, NEW YORK

AVAILABLE ONLY THROUGH YOUR AVON REPRESENTATIVE WHO CALLS AT YOUR HOME

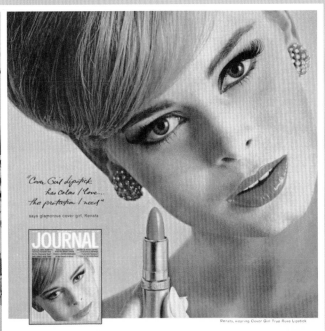

"Cover Girl lipstick has colors I love . . . the protection I need" says glamorous cover girl, Renata

JOURNAL

Renata, wearing Cover Girl True Rose Lipstick

New! Glamour that's good for your lips—Cover Girl Lipstick!

First lipstick with beautiful colors chosen by cover girls . . . plus beautifying medication. Helps lips stay cover girl smooth, moist, luscious!

It's the most completely beautifying lipstick ever. All the right colors! And for the first time, the protection you've always wanted from dryness. Beautifying medication by Noxzema helps keep lips soft, moist . . . with no medicated taste or odor. It's glamour that's good for your lips.

Your lips look better, feel better than ever before—with Cover Girl Medicated Lipstick. So keep your lips cover girl luscious. Get fragrant Cover Girl Lipstick. Better yet, get two or three. Then create your own "custom-mixed" colors. That's just what the beautiful cover girls do.

COVER GIRL MEDICATED LIPSTICK BY NOXZEMA

POW! cover girl ignites the glitter explosion

WOW! the 'SHINERS' are here!

Five shiny-sheer new lip shades make the sheen-scene! (It's the new-and-now look that glows with the new-and-now glitter clothes!) Translucent, but there. Hot, but bare. Positively super-silvered. It's your time to shine, baby. And the 'Shiners' are here!

COVER GIRL
MEDICATED LIPSTICKS
BY NOXZEMA

GLAZED ORANGE

LILAC FROST

CRANBERRY ICE

WHITE-HOT SILVER

PINK-HOT SILVER

(Two brilliant new sizzle sticks that zing up any color!)

CoverGirl brand shiny-sheer lipstick advertisement, 1966.

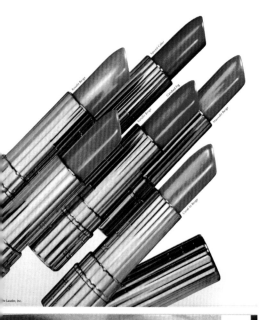

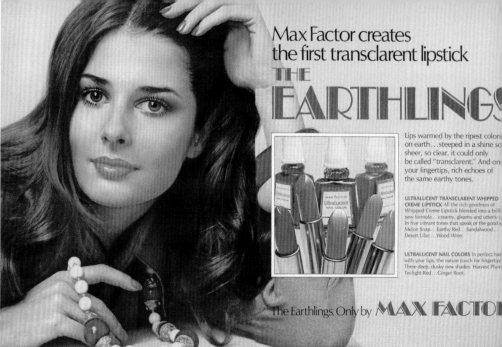

Max Factor creates
the first transclarent lipstick

THE EARTHLINGS

Lips warmed by the ripest colors on earth...steeped in a shine so sheer, so clear, it could only be called "transclarent." And on your fingertips, rich echoes of the same earthy tones.

ULTRALUCENT TRANSCLARENT WHIPPED CREME LIPSTICK All the rich goodness of Whipped Creme Lipstick blended into a brilliant new formula...creamy, gleamy and utterly c In five vibrant tones that speak of the good e Melon Snap... Earthy Red... Sandalwood... Desert Lilac... Wood Wine.

ULTRALUCENT NAIL COLORS In perfect har with your lips, the nature touch for fingertips Three deep, dusky new shades: Harvest Plum Twilight Red...Ginger Root.

The Earthlings. Only by **MAX FACTOR**

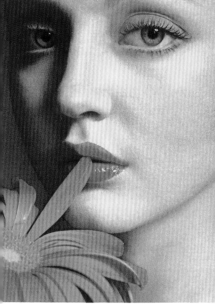

THIS IS LOVE IN 1972

New Lovestick Color Glazes.
You can't get this kind of clear, fresh-picked lip color anywhere else.

New Lovestick Color Glazes™ are different than lipstick or gloss. Lovestick Color Glazes are almost transparent. Their colors are rich and vibrant and clean on your mouth. And they have just enough shine to give you a look as fresh and moist as the flowers of spring.

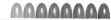

PINK GLAZE PEACH GLAZE TOMATO GLAZE RED GLAZE RASPBERRY GLAZE COPPER GLAZE CRANBERRY GLAZE WALNUT GLAZE

Love Cosmetics by Menley & James.

Clockwise from top left:

Estée Lauder brand lipsticks in Cool Sand Beige colors, 1984.

Max Factor brand Earthlings lipstick advertisement, 1972.

CoverGirl brand Lip Blush lipstick advertisement, model Cheryl Tiegs, 1982.

Love Cosmetics by Menley & James brand Lovestick Color Glaze lipstick advertisement, 1972.

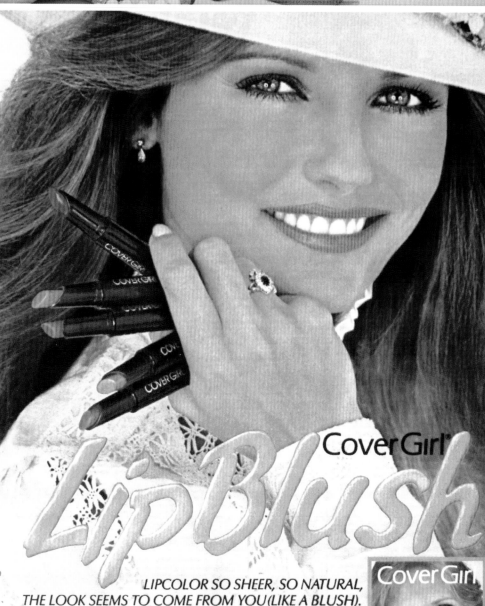

Cover Girl® *LipBlush*

LIPCOLOR SO SHEER, SO NATURAL, THE LOOK SEEMS TO COME FROM YOU (LIKE A BLUSH).

It's color and shine that look so natural, feel so fresh, Cover Girl® had to call it LipBlush. Cover Girl LipBlush. Specially formulated for a longer, slimmer case with a professional slant tip for mistake-proof shaping and defining. So color glides on smoothly, evenly-stays sheer. Cover Girl LipBlush. In 14 innocent shades.

Cover Girl Cheryl Tiegs is wearing Shellpink LipBlush.

Cover Girl

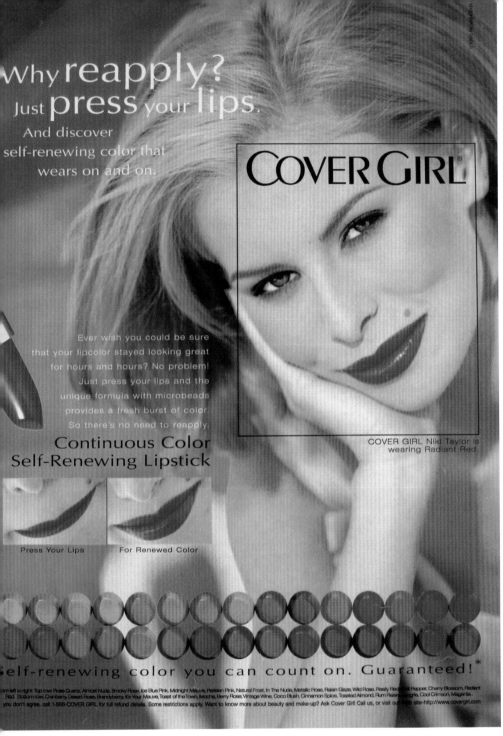

CoverGirl brand Continuous Color Self-Renewing Lipstick advertisement, model Niki Taylor, 1996.

Natural formulas were created in the 1990s using oils such as jojoba, castor, coconut, rosehip, and sunflower. Other products used cocoa or shea butter, Beeswax, grapefruit, strawberry, or cherry extracts. Due to their new formulas, lipsticks were now softer compared to the hard and waxy lipsticks beforehand, and because they used plant-based colorants, the pigments were sheer and not as deep or bright.

By the end of the '90s and well into the first decade of the new millennium, a lipstick's purpose has taken on more than adding color to the lips. Lipsticks added lip plumping ingredients, collagen, vitamins, sunscreen, and other cosmeceutical ingredients to keep lips healthy, soft, and sensuous.

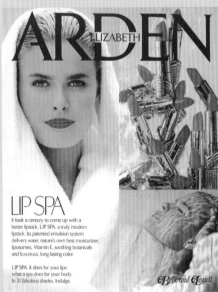

Elizabeth Arden brand Lip Spa lipstick advertisement, 1992.

In 2000, the staying power of lipsticks improved. Lipstick formulations that previously smudged and feathered became practically permanent on the lips. Max Factor launched Lipfinity, a liquid lipstick that was painted on, then sealed with a separate top coat. It contained Perma Tone, a semi-permanent color that had eight hours of continuous wear. In the Autumn of 2005, Maybelline launched Superstay lipstick with a similar two-system format as Lipfinity.

For the savvy consumer looking to spotlight one of the most provocative parts of the female body, the options in lipstick choices are endless with regard to texture, shine, and ingredients. Because lipstick is arguably the favorite and most popular cosmetic product among women today, hundreds of patents for lipstick dispensers and innovative formulations exist and will continue to be filed.

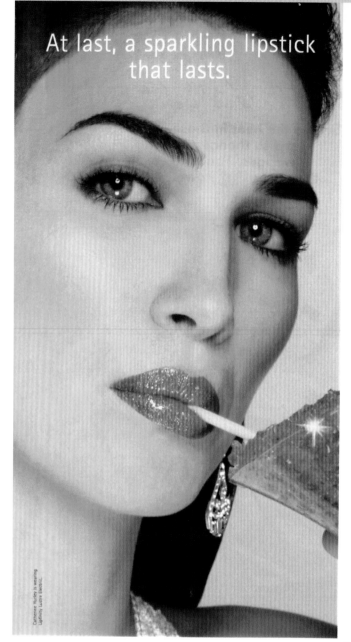

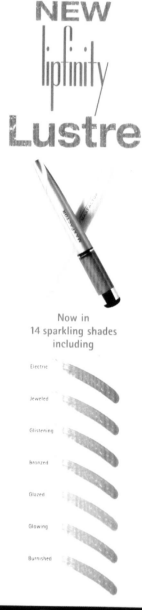

Max Factor brand Lipfinity lipstick advertisement, 2003.

The Face

Attention to aging skin has been a priority for over 3000 years. In ancient times, masks were used to cleanse and maintain the skin's moisture. The Egyptians used anti-wrinkle creams made with the essential oil of frankincense, which claimed to possess anti-inflammatory properties. Thick creams, created to preserve moisture on mature skin, were formulated from resin, wax, oil, grass, and plant juice. A milk bath, supposedly one of Cleopatra's favorite indulgences, was believed to keep the skin clear because the lactic acid in the milk had the effect of a peel as it got rid of dead skin cells and revealed a healthy new layer of skin.

Scrubs were widely used during Roman times to refine the skin's texture. These were fashioned from seeds, orris root, and honey. Face packs made with starch and eggs were believed to tighten the skin and keep it youthful. Some women used crocodile dung to preserve their complexion.

During Medieval times, herbs and salves were used to guard the skin against the cold. Soap was used as a medicinal aid rather than as a daily cleanser.

The Middle Ages brought the practice of creating cosmetic aids within the home. Women made white face makeup from wheat. Castile soap was used as fine toilette soap by the wealthy.

The sixteenth and seventeenth centuries brought many "cures" for freckles and a flood of miracle face creams. Toners made from oil of bay, rhubarb, spices, and wine were sold by traveling salesmen. Lemon juice and eggs were used as a face mask, and egg whites were used as foundation for a taut and shiny complexion. Other home remedies included concoctions to alleviate chapped hands and lighten face spots. Facial cleansing creams were made from soft soap mixed with abrasives or astringents. Sugar, borax, and camphor were popular ingredients for these creams, which exfoliated the skin and dried up blemishes.

The eighteenth century marked the use of scented waters and face toners. Cold cream made with scented oils, spermaceti, and wax, then mixed with rosewater and ambergris, was a common toilette preparation. Other skin products made at home included skin lighteners composed of alum and egg whites, and a facial cream called Eau de Veau made from boiled calf's foot. Most skin preparations required cold storage to avoid spoilage because they included animal fats. Oils in these preparations quickly turned rancid once applied to the skin.

Acid peels were common in the late 1870s, and the phenol peel, performed with carbonic acid, was believed to restore softness to the skin. By 1880, peels known as skinning were practiced in salons and unregulated private homes.

During the nineteenth and twentieth centuries, mass produced products became available to women for purchase. Harriet Hubbard Ayer was one of the first to promote her commercial face cream with the help of actress Lillie Langtry. Helena Rubinstein marketed her cream from her mother's recipe in Poland. The Pond's Company produced a commercially successful vanishing cream with the innovation of a mineral oil base that resisted spoilage. The 1920s brought an increased fascination with youth popularized by lively flappers, and cosmetic companies were quick to deliver innovative sales pitches to guarantee a youthful look.

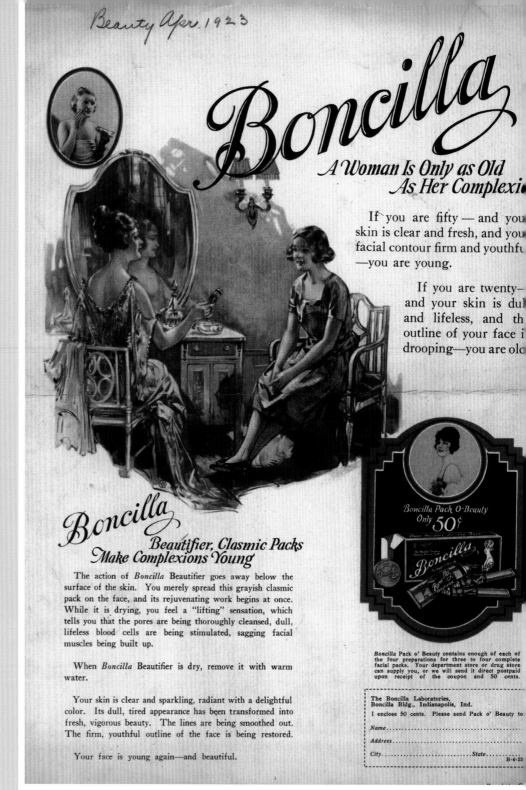

Boncilla Beautifier cream advertisement, 1923.

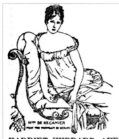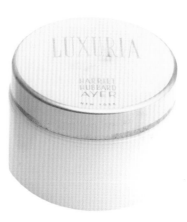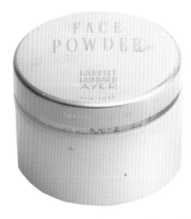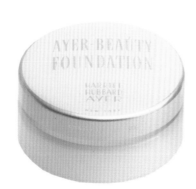

RÉCAMIER CREAM
FOR THE COMPLEXION

Has been in use for nearly a century. It was originally made for the most celebrated beauty of her time—Madame JULIE RÉCAMIER—and by its constant use she retained her exquisite complexion until her death, at eighty.

RÉCAMIER CREAM is the only preparation of its kind which has received the indorsements of eminent physicians and chemists. Used by Her Royal Highness the Princess of Wales, Mesdames Adelina Patti, Sarah Bernhardt, James Brown Potter, Langtry, Lillian Russell, and thousands of fashionable women all over the world.

RÉCAMIER CREAM is not a cosmetic. You apply it at night and wash it off in the morning.

Price $1.50 per Jar. Sample bottle sent postpaid on receipt of 25 Cents.

HARRIET HUBBARD AYER, Recamier Mfg Co., 131 W. 31st St., New York.

Harriet Hubbard Ayer Recamier Cream advertisement, c. late 1890s.

Harriet Hubbard Ayer Makeup Caddy set with face powder, foundation, and cream, 1930.

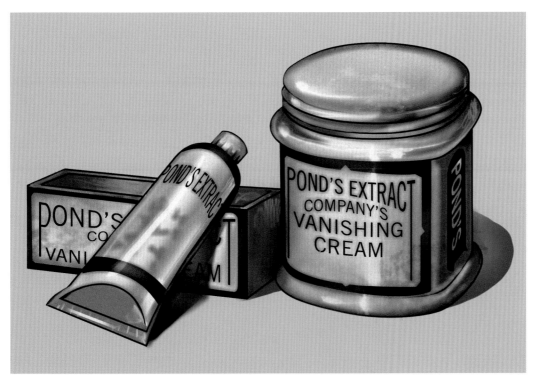

Pond's Vanishing Cream, 1915.

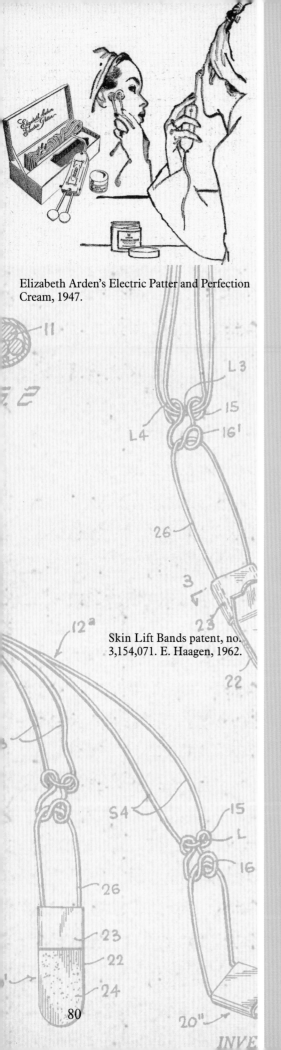

Elizabeth Arden's Electric Patter and Perfection Cream, 1947.

Skin Lift Bands patent, no. 3,154,071. E. Haagen, 1962.

The advent of electricity extended to the cosmetic arts, and by 1930, electrical current with pulsating microwaves was used by salons for facial treatments to tighten and restore the skin. Many machines were invented for this purpose, including the Violet Ray machine that advertised it would "increase secretions" and "soothe the nervous system."

Other salon procedures created to improve the skin included the Arden Youth Mask, which consisted of a paper mask with tin foil connected to a box that supplied low levels of microwave energy. A hot-wax bath called the Ardena Bath, involved being painted with a hot wax mixture and wrapped in paraffin paper to rid the body of impurities and poisons.

In the early 1900s, the face-lift was performed with local anesthesia, but without the use of antibiotics; it often resulted in infections to the wounds. Other temporary lifting options, such as the Hollywood Lift, included various contraptions that secured the skin with rubber bands, glue, and thread.

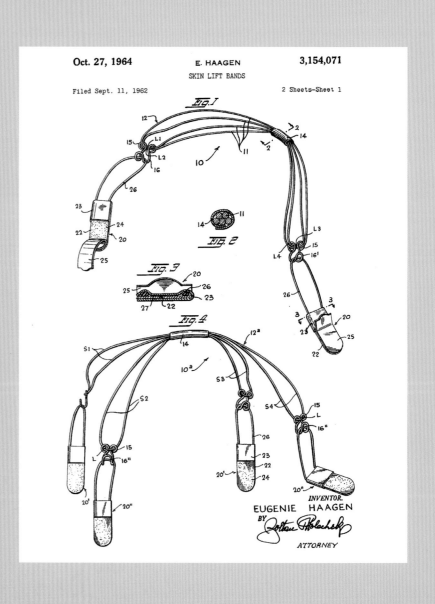

By the late 1950s, surgical techniques improved, and modern drugs were used to make the procedures safer and more effective. Celebrities were the first to adopt the procedures, followed by the society crowd. By the 1960s, surgery was an option for the middle class and became acceptable by the housewife in the pursuit of perfection.

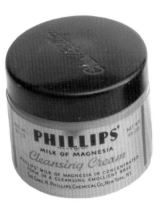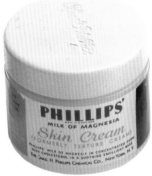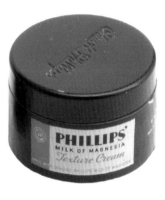

Phillips' Milk of Magnesia Cleansing Cream, Skin Cream, and Texture Cream, in white glass jars with metal lids, c. late 1930s.

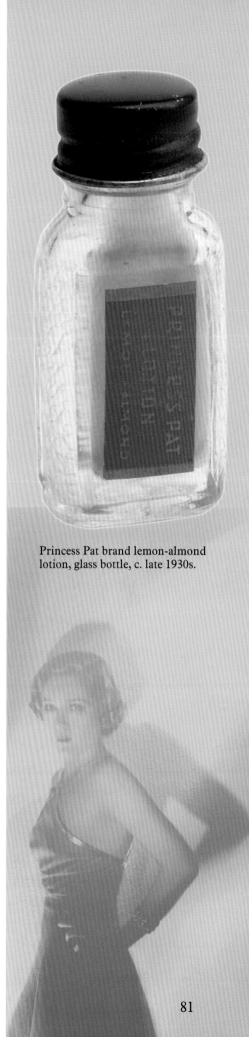

Princess Pat brand lemon-almond lotion, glass bottle, c. late 1930s.

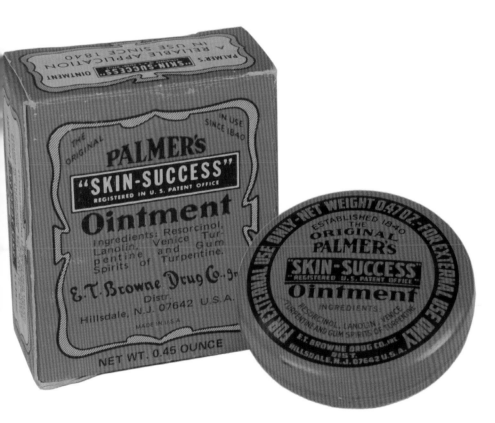

Palmer's "Skin-Success" Ointment, c. 1940.

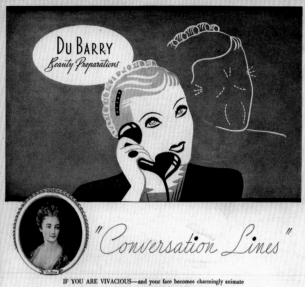

DuBarry

Beauty Preparations

"Conversation Lines"

IF YOU ARE VIVACIOUS—and your face becomes charmingly animate when you talk—guard against conversation lines! First, a thorough cleansing with Du Barry Liquefying Cleansing Cream and Du Barry Skin Tonic and Freshener. Then, a generous mask of Du Barry Special Skin Food over face and throat—a film of Du Barry Muscle Oil over expression lines. Try this tonight! You'll delight in the smoothness, the softness of your skin after this treatment. Ask any fine shop for Du Barry Skin Food, 1.50, 2.50, 4.50; Du Barry Muscle Oil, 1.00, 1.50, 2.50; Du Barry Cleansing Cream, 1.00, 1.50, 2.50, 4.50; Du Barry Skin Tonic & Freshener, 1.00, 1.75, 3.50.

★ ★ ★ ★

IT'S THE TOP... The newly opened Sports Roof of the Richard Hudnut Salon, Six Nine Three Fifth Avenue, is a Four-Star Success! It is the crowning glory of the only salon in the world that offers a complete regime of beauty, health and slenderness under one roof... *and what a roof!*
ANN DELAFIELD DIRECTING.

New York **RICHARD HUDNUT** *Paris*

DuBarry Beauty Preparations advertisement, c. 1940s.

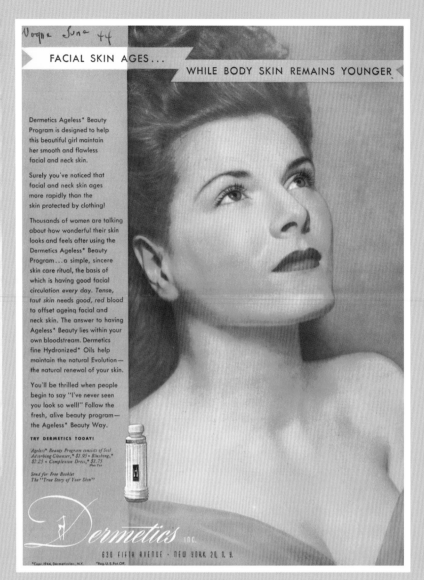

FACIAL SKIN AGES...

Vogue June 44

WHILE BODY SKIN REMAINS YOUNGER

Dermetics Ageless* Beauty Program is designed to help this beautiful girl maintain her smooth and flawless facial and neck skin.

Surely you've noticed that facial and neck skin ages more rapidly than the skin protected by clothing!

Thousands of women are talking about how wonderful their skin looks and feels after using the Dermetics Ageless* Beauty Program...a simple, sincere skin care ritual, the basis of which is having good facial circulation every day. Tense, taut skin needs good, red blood to offset ageing facial and neck skin. The answer to having Ageless* Beauty lies within your own bloodstream. Dermetics fine Hydronized* Oils help maintain the natural Evolution — the natural renewal of your skin.

You'll be thrilled when people begin to say "I've never seen you look so well!" Follow the fresh, alive beauty program— the Ageless* Beauty Way.

TRY DERMETICS TODAY!

Ageless Beauty Program consists of Seal Adsorbing Cleanser,* $1.95 • Blushing,* $2.25 • Complexion Dress,* $1.75 Plus Tax*

Send for Free Booklet The "True Story of Your Skin"

Dermetics INC.

630 FIFTH AVENUE · NEW YORK 20, N. Y.

*Copr. 1944, Dermetics Inc., N.Y.   *Reg. U.S. Pat. Off.

Dermetics Ageless Beauty Program advertisement, 1944.

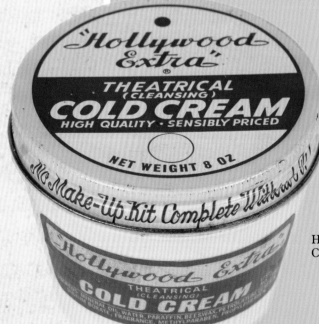

Hollywood Extra brand Theatrical Cleansing Cold Cream, 1939.

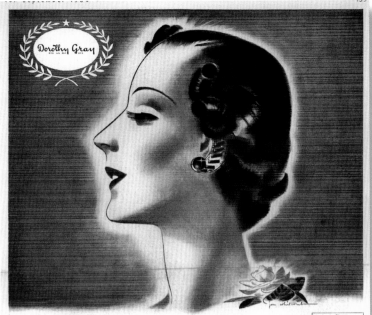

The "peaches and cream" complexion was the basis of all 1950s skincare trends. In order to prevail in the skincare market, foundations and pressed powders had to promote a soft, feminine look. Palmolive bars were sold as effective skin cleansers. Noxzema cold cream contained camphor, menthol, and eucalyptus to give off a refreshing, tingling feeling. Its main competitor was Albolene. These products were popular among women as facial cleansers and makeup removers. Creams from Pond's contained lanolin as the main moisturizer, a yellow waxy substance secreted by the sebaceous glands of sheep.

Dorothy Gray creams advertisement, 1936.

DuBarry Beauty-Angle Treatment advertisement, 1937.

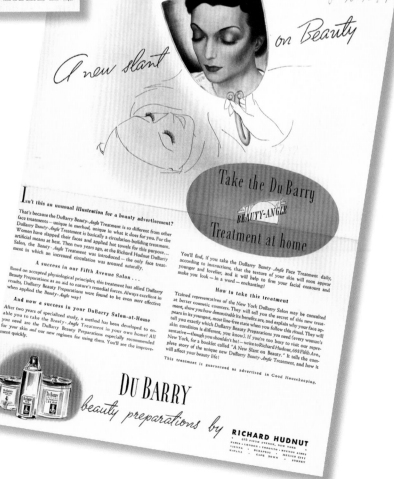

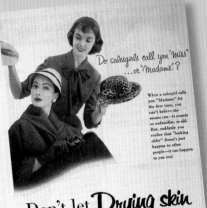

Pond's Dry Skin Cream
advertisement, 1956.

Will you look as youthful as Gloria Swanson at 53 ?

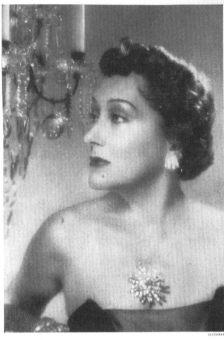

Don't let **Drying skin** "middle-age" your face

It can happen even before 25—the dreaded "older" look of dry skin. Tired little crow's feet . . . rough, flaky patches . . . tiny dry lines—all these tell you that your skin's natural softening oils are beginning to dry out. *By 40, the skin can actually lose up to 20% of its own softening oil.* So, to prevent the "middle-aging" effects of dry skin, you must *replace* these oils *every day!*

You can't expect a thin liquid to do the work of a rich cream

Parched, dried-out skin needs more than surface oiling with a thin, runny liquid. Dry skin needs the *deep-softening* benefits of a full-textured, quick-penetrating, rich cream.

Today's leading dry skin care—Pond's Dry Skin Cream—has three special features that make it an unusually effective dry skin treatment.

1. **It's extra rich in lanolin**, the oil most like your own natural skin softeners.
2. **Homogenized lanolin.** The lanolin in Pond's Dry Skin Cream is not ordinary

lanolin—it's homogenized into tiny particles that penetrate almost instantly.
3. **Its special emulsifier** restores "dewiness" to flaky, dried-out surface skin.

Tonight—start to use rich, deep-softening Pond's Dry Skin Cream. See how much softer, fresher, and younger your skin soon looks!

How to solve these dry skin problems

Dry crow's feet around eyes make you look tired, older. To deep-soften —gently tap in silky, quick-penetrating Pond's Dry Skin Cream.

Dry flaky roughness coarsens skin texture, spoils your make-up. To *smooth away*—apply this lanolin-rich cream with brisk little circling motions.

Dry crinkle lines on forehead and throat look "matronly." To ease out—smooth Pond's Dry Skin Cream upward and outward on forehead, upward on throat. See dry skin "drink up" the cream's lanolin-richness.

Get your Pond's Dry Skin Cream *today* in the large jar—a whole season's supply for less than one dollar!

Extra Rich in Lanolin

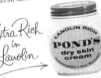

So effective— more women use it than any other dry skin care

January 1956

"After all," Gloria Swanson smiled, "I don't *live* by flattering candlelight! So thank goodness I've found *one simple care* that holds *all* the secrets of youthful-looking skin — JERGENS ALL-PURPOSE FACE CREAM!"

Jergens Cream, made with wonderful VITONE, is a really *thorough* cleanser. Its superfine oils loosen every particle of dirt and stale cosmetics — leave your skin exquisitely, radiantly clean.

It's an effective lubricant, too. Vitone helps supplement the natural oils you tend to lose with age, and helps smooth away little dry lines.

And it's the ideal powder base, because Vitone continues its smoothing action while Jergens Cream makes your powder cling with peach-bloom softness.

Jergens Cream is *three* beauty creams in one. So use it faithfully every day and be one of those enchanting women who looks years younger than she is!

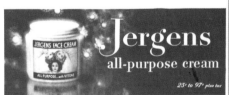

Jergens
all-purpose cream

25¢ to 97¢ plus tax

ENRICHED WITH PRECIOUS **VITONE**!

22

Jergens All-Purpose Face Cream advertisement, featuring Gloria Swanson, 1952.

Avon brand cosmetics
Cleansing Creams
advertisement, 1947.

AVON ANNOUNCES
2 NEW CLEANSING CREAMS

For a lovelier skin

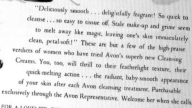

"Deliciously smooth . . . delightfully fragrant! So quick to cleanse . . . so easy to tissue off. Stale make-up and grime seem to melt away like magic, leaving one's skin immaculately clean, petal-soft!" These are but a few of the high-praise verdicts of women who have tried Avon's superb new Cleansing Creams. You, too, will thrill to their featherlight texture, their quick-melting action . . . the radiant, baby-smooth appearance of your skin after each Avon cleansing treatment. Purchasable exclusively through the Avon Representative. Welcome her when she calls.

FOR A LOVELIER SKIN . . . USE AVON'S NEW CLEANSING CREAMS

Avon Cleansing Cream (Creamy)
Whipped-cream light, satin-smooth, quick-melting, this new Avon Cleansing Cream is perfect for all types of skin . . . a "must" for dry skin.

Avon Cleansing Cream (Liquefying)
New, improved formula. Softer, quicker-melting, thoroughly-cleansing. Suits all types of skin —excellent for oily skin.

Avon Skin Freshener or Astringent
Use after each cleansing to remove every trace of cream, insure a scrupulously clean skin, keep it firmer, finer-textured, stimulate a fresher color.

Avon __cosmetics

IN RADIO CITY, NEW YORK

84

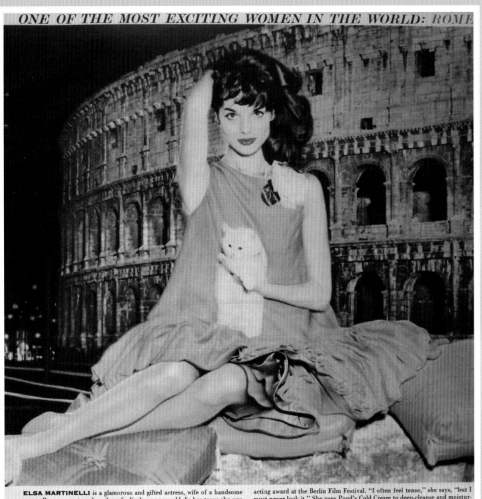

ELSA MARTINELLI is a glamorous and gifted actress, wife of a handsome young Roman count, and mother of a lively one-year-old. In her teens she was a top-flight fashion model in Paris and New York. Recently she won the top acting award at the Berlin Film Festival. "I often feel tense," she says, "but I must never look it." She uses Pond's Cold Cream to deep-cleanse and moisturize . . . to ease away tension lines . . . "My skin stays soft and smooth all day long."

She's busy...
yet she's beautiful...
she uses Pond's

ELSA MARTINELLI says: "Pond's beautifies as it cleanses!" Yes, this fabulous cream deep-moisturizes as it cleanses and freshens every tiny pore. And this richer cream goes on moisturizing long after you tissue it off. "Plumps up" the skin cells so tired lines can smooth out. Your skin will stay soft and smooth. See it come alive and glow with an exciting new beauty—like Elsa Martinelli's Use Pond's Cold Cream to beauty-cleanse at night to moisturize under make-up all day.

NOW! POND'S COLD CREAM IN STUNNING NEW DESIGNER JAR!

Pond's Cold Cream advertisement, 1960.

Multi-step skincare systems arrived in the 1960s. Regimens included moisturizers, toners, and cleansers. Elizabeth Arden's Eight Hour Cream contained vitamin E and was one of the first products to use petrolatum, a skin-soothing beta-hydroxy. Tussy Medicare was a three-step kit for combating pimples. It contained a deep cleansing mask, a toner, and a medicated lotion.

The 1970s saw "natural" ingredients being incorporated into cosmetics to satisfy the growing need for organic products. Clinique emerged as a brand with an image of scientific authority. Their white makeup counters were attended by white-coated employees. More skincare products were developed for the ethnic market and for the men's sector.

Revlon brand Moon Drops Under Makeup Moisture Film advertisement, 1976.

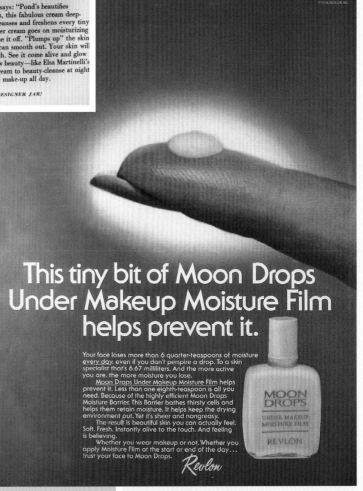

This tiny bit of Moon Drops Under Makeup Moisture Film helps prevent it.

Your face loses more than 6 quarter-teaspoons of moisture every day, even if you don't perspire a drop. To a skin specialist that's 6.67 milliliters. And the more active you are, the more moisture you lose.

Moon Drops Under Makeup Moisture Film helps prevent it. Less than one eighth-teaspoon is all you need. Because of the highly efficient Moon Drops Moisture Barrier. This Barrier bathes thirsty cells and helps them retain moisture. It helps keep the drying environment out. Yet it's sheer and nongreasy.

The result is beautiful skin you can actually feel. Soft. Fresh. Instantly alive to the touch. And feeling is believing.

Whether you wear makeup or not. Whether you apply Moisture Film at the start or end of the day... trust your face to Moon Drops.

Revlon

MOON DROPS
UNDER MAKEUP
MOISTURE FILM
REVLON

By the 1980s, collagen and other extracts were used in skin formulas. The first anti-aging skincare products appeared during the late 1980s. A liposome ingredient delivery system was used in the first generation of anti-aging skincare products. These products were marketed to firm up, soften the skin, and reduce lines.

Revlon brand European Collagen Complex beauty cream advertisement, 1984.

Estée Lauder brand Swiss Performing Extract lotion advertisement, 1986.

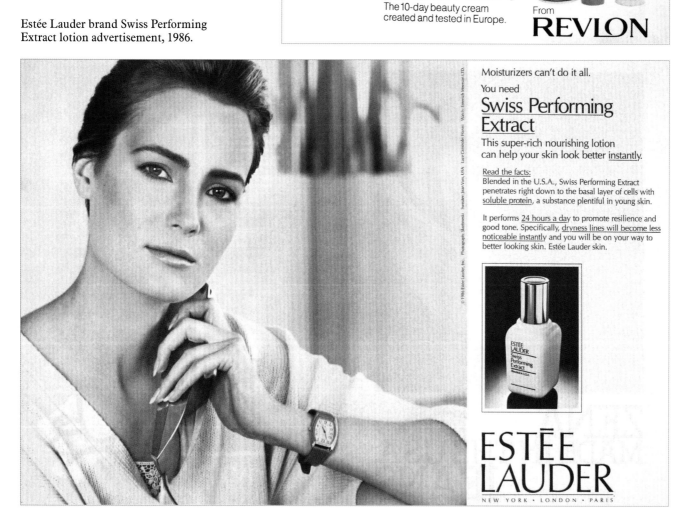

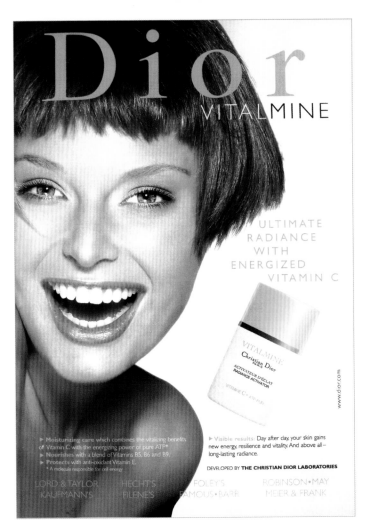

Christian Dior brand Vitalmine
moisturizer, advertisement, 1999.

The 1990s brought in the use of vitamins and other ingredients to moisturize and protect the skin. The most important of those, Alpha Hydroxyl Acids (AHA), became the first ingredient to affect aging skin. The role of vitamins A, C, and E, as well as group B vitamins and main fatty acids were discovered to have a special role in preventing premature aging.

Revlon brand Eterna '27' night cream,
model Lauren Hutton, 1991.

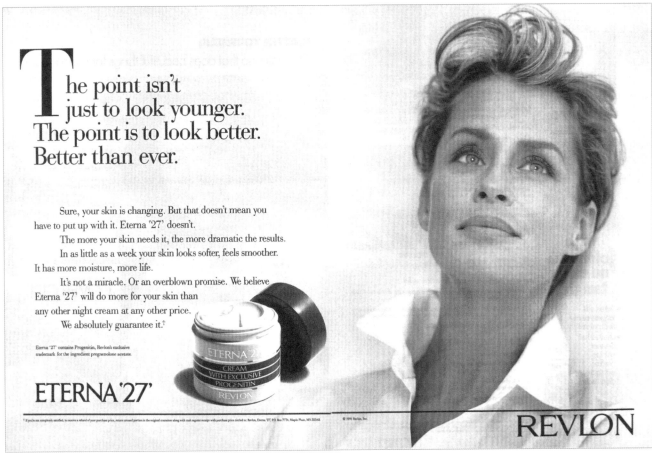

By the 2000s, formulas included retinols, hyaluronic acids as effective skin moisturizers, and nano particles that could penetrate deeply into the skin to slow down aging and protect skin cells. Manufacturers started using anti-oxidants, sunscreens, and skin energizing technologies to "recharge" cells. Described as the next generation of skin nourishers, they enabled skin to rebuild itself and retain a youthful appearance. Chemists in the cosmetics field have noted these changes. Fred H. Khoury, an independent research and development chemist, states that the cosmetics industry has made a dramatic movement away from animal and synthetic ingredients to the incorporation of all or partial amounts of vegan and organic ingredients in skin, hair care, and color cosmetics. He also notes that creams previously featuring steroid hormones such as progesterone, estrogen, and placental extracts have made way to serums containing peptides and botanical stem cell cultured extracts.

With today's technological advances in new compounds to keep skin youthful, creams and miracle potions are released at great speed to women who are constantly looking for ways to stall the passage of time. Women today have hundreds of choices in the types of treatments and products best suited to maintain the skin. They look to the near future for the next best thing that holds the promise of eternal youth.

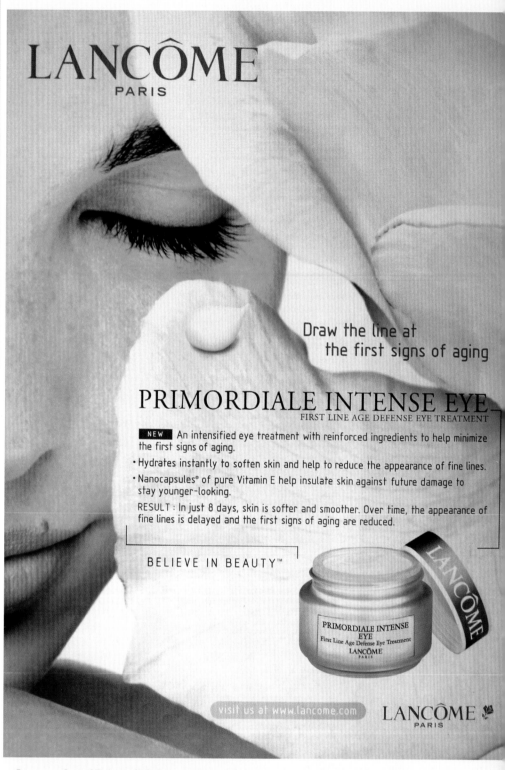

Lancome brand Primordiale Intense Eye – First Line Age Defense Eye Treatment advertisement, 2000.

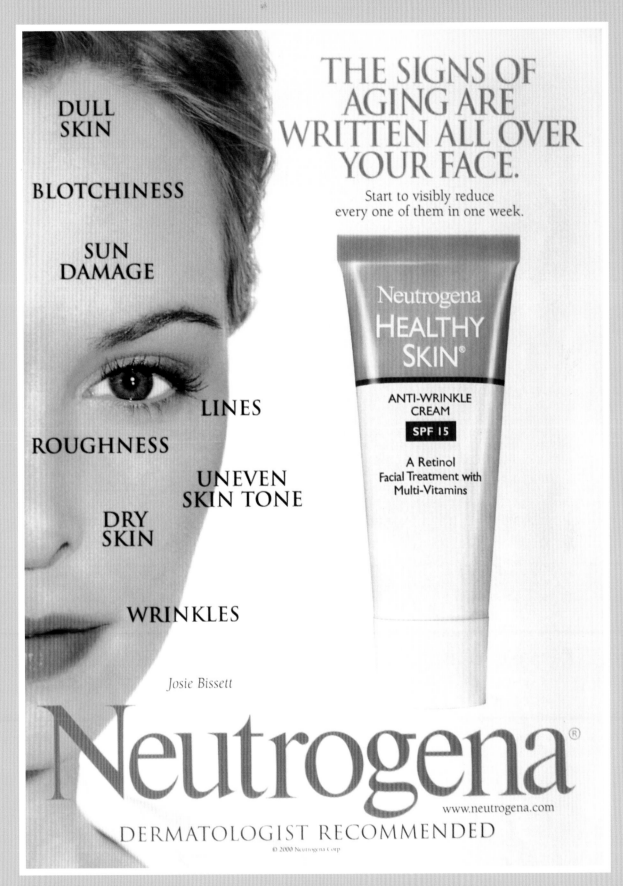

Neutrogena brand Healthy Skin anti-wrinkle cream with SPF 15, advertisement, 2000.

Historical TIMELINE

A.D. 1920 to A.D. 1929

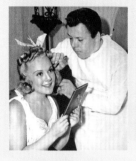

Perc Westmore, makeup director at Warner Bros. Studios, establishes Westmore Cosmetics in Hollywood. Westmore pictured with actress Sonja Henie.

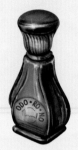

Edna Murphey Albert expands her door-to-door deodorant sales and establishes the Odorono Company.

Sara Spencer Washington establishes the Apex Hair and News Company. It becomes one of the largest African American owned businesses during the 1920s and '30s.

M. Martin Gordon and his wife Frances Patricia Berry establish Princess Pat cosmetics brand. Known as the Beauty Editors of the airwaves, they do lectures on cosmetics and advertise their brand during radio broadcasts.

1920
The general acceptance of beauty preparations leads to the development of many brands of products. Soap, perfume, cold cream, vanishing cream, eye shadow, rouge, and face powder are some of the most popular items.

Dorothy Gray, Marie Earle, and Kathleen Mary Quinlan establish factories to sell their brands of cosmetic products.

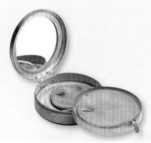

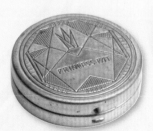

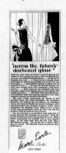

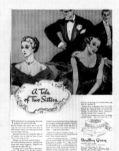

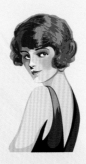

1926
Young flappers use heavy dark red lipstick and penciled-in eyebrows to stand out and shock their parents. Eventually, the look catches on and the mothers adopt the makeup and fashion trends of their daughters.

1929
Carl Weeks launches Florian, a line of men's products that includes skin lotion, face powder, and moisturizer.

1925
The cosmetics industry grows to 1 billion per year.

1928
Madame Mille's manicure shop in Paris popularizes the "moon manicure," which leaves the tips and moons of the nails white.

Tanning lotion and darker face powder enter the market as darker skin becomes fashionable.

Women's emancipation inspires a wider use of cosmetic products and the practice of applying makeup in public with brushes and powder puffs.

1922
Elizabeth Arden opens her cosmetics salon in France.

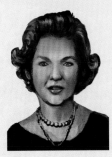

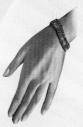

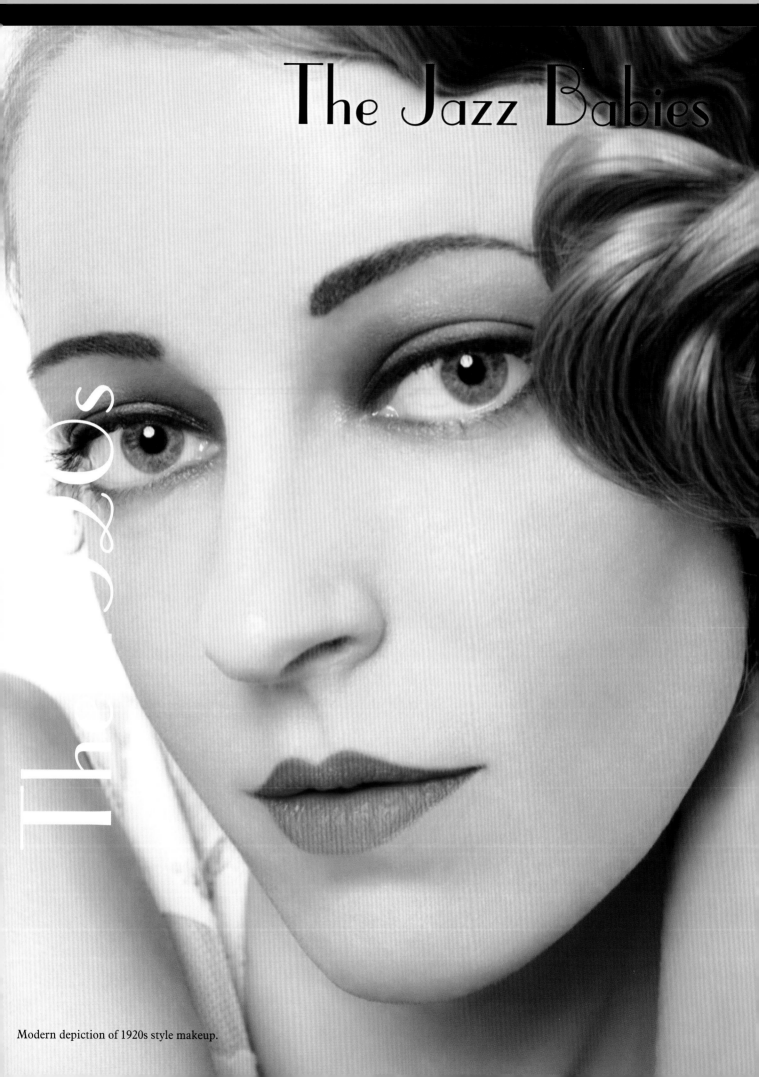

The Jazz Babies

The 1920s

Modern depiction of 1920s style makeup.

Fueled by the Suffrage movement and the advent of the modern woman, the 1920s marked a resurgence in the use of makeup by women. With a newly designed twist-up tube of lipstick, it was considered chic to apply makeup in public. Advertising appealed to a woman's insecurities by marketing solutions for beauty dilemmas. Cosmetics made a woman believe that she would achieve natural loveliness and look her most attractive with its usage. Rebelliousness defined the era, launched by the women's vote but scandalized by the Prohibition Act, adding the naughtiness of speakeasies and bathtub gin to the giddy equation.

Any woman concerned with fashion wore makeup. The look was far from subtle. The face was layered with powder and strong rouge. The eyebrows were plucked thin. The eyes were rimmed with black kohl, and bright heavy shadows colored the eyelids. The lips were painted dark red and outlined in two small mounds to form the perfect bee-stung lips. The ideal color complexion was pale. It started with cream and ivory in the beginning of the decade followed by peach and more natural shades by the late '20s.

Lipstick use was on the rise as dark red shades became the standard color for the flapper. Flappers got their name from the unbuckled boots they oftern wore with simple chemise dresses, rouged knees, and bobbed hair. Her favorite accessory was the tango case, a compact used as a purse that contained powder, rouge, lipstick, and a card or cigarette compartment.

As a sign of modernity and independence, many women adopted a bobbed hairstyle with a finger wave called the Eton crop. The style was made popular by the invention of the Marcel wave created with a hot rounded iron. Cutting their hair was a big decision for women and proved unfavorable with men who wanted women to retain the image of a wholesome Gibson girl. Working in factories as part of the war effort made the tedious task of styling long hair a nuisance. As the supply of eligible men dwindled after the war, bachelorettes moved away from their families and attempted to support themselves. They needed an easier routine and gravitated to shorter hairstyles and simple dresses. The popularity of the cloche hat complemented short hairstyles. A large portion of the money young women earned was used to purchase clothing and cosmetics.

Young women emulated the styles of their favorite on-screen actresses of the day, which included Gloria Swanson, Pola Negri, and Clara Bow. These seductive screen sirens replaced the society women who had inspired fashion and style before the war. With the help of Max Factor, actresses were groomed to perfection with new greaseless paints that looked more natural on film. He manufactured a society line of products endorsed by his Hollywood actress clientele. Factor also introduced the idea of matching colors for lips, cheeks, and powder.

Black entertainers of the time, such as Josephine Baker, brought exoticism, black beauty, and an appreciation for all things African to the forefront. Baker used egg whites to shine her hair and white pencil around the inner lash-line to create the illusion of larger eyes. In productions like *Revue Negre*, Baker was often clad only in a skirt made of bananas. This style of exotic spectacle remained popular decades later when jazz great Billie Holiday appeared covered in orchids.

With the popularity of black beauty and the invention of suntan oil by the end of the decade, darker skin became popular during the summer months. Coco Chanel is widely credited with popularizing the suntan, following a French Riviera vacation—a vibrant change from pallor mortis. Cosmetics responded with darker hued powders and lighter lip colors to contrast dark suntanned skin. However, women were encouraged to have a white and pale complexion during the winter.

The popular vamp look required women to wear binding fashions that flattened the chest. Women adopted diets to conform to these slim styles. The typical woman wore a tank top dress with a low waist and a chemise. Legs were left bare, and the most popular shoes were the Louis heel or the ankle strap Mary Jane. The use of Rayon fabrics made maintenance simple and provided affordability for the local manufacturing of fashions.

The 1920s marked the beginning of the pursuit of youth. Mature women were never again seen to be truly fashionable. Women strived to look young, for youth was now synonymous with beauty. Cosmetics such as wrinkle reducers, restorers, and youth creams were invented to help preserve a fresh and youthful look.

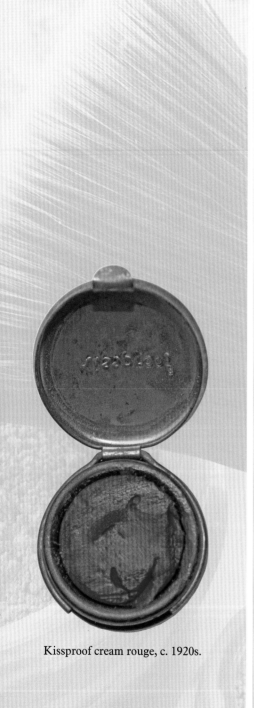

Kissproof cream rouge, c. 1920s.

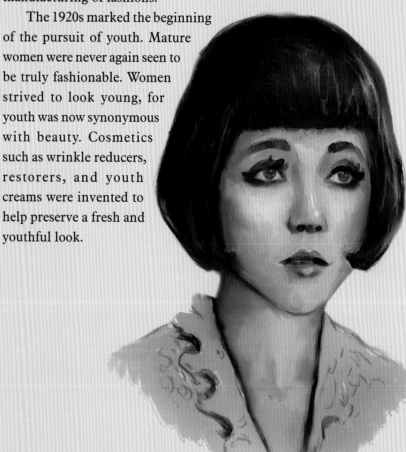

Decade Highlights

- National advertising establishes ties between cosmetic manufacturers and mass media through magazines, movies, and fashion.
- Stores begin to use point of purchase promotions. They place movie stills next to the products and design mannequins to look like the popular screen sirens.
- Advertising features movie stars such as Mary Pickford for Pompeian Beauty.
- Elizabeth Arden sales representatives are one of the first to educate women on the use of complete lines of products designed to work together.
- To encourage sales, department stores sponsor beauty weeks with lectures, makeup lessons, and free samples.
- Cosmetics are available to the masses with the growth of the chain store started by the five and ten stores.
- As competition flourishes, artists are commissioned to create distinctive boxes and bottles. Powder compacts and lipstick cartridges become major fashion accessories.
- The discovery of Tutankhamun's tomb popularizes the Egyptian look.
- Kurlash eyelash curlers and "612" mascara produced by Pinaud appear on the market.
- Max Factor receives an Academy Award for his Panchromatic Foundation, the first for a makeup product.
- It is the beginning of the popularity for tanned skin and a fascination with African culture.
- The first nail polish in sheer red and the French manicure look are introduced.
- Chanel No. 5 introduces synthetic perfume ingredients.
- "We adore makeup and the gilded lily, and why not?" Cecil Beaton, 1928.

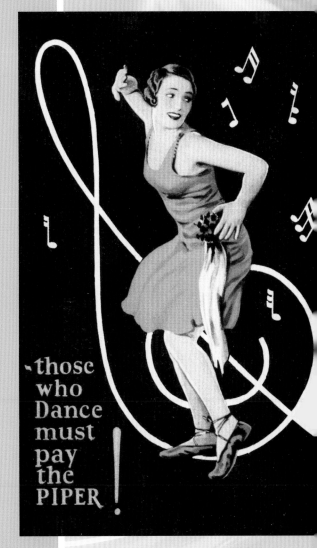

Dance Magic, cover of the publicity brochure for the 1927 silent movie about life in the Broadway musical theatre.

The Face

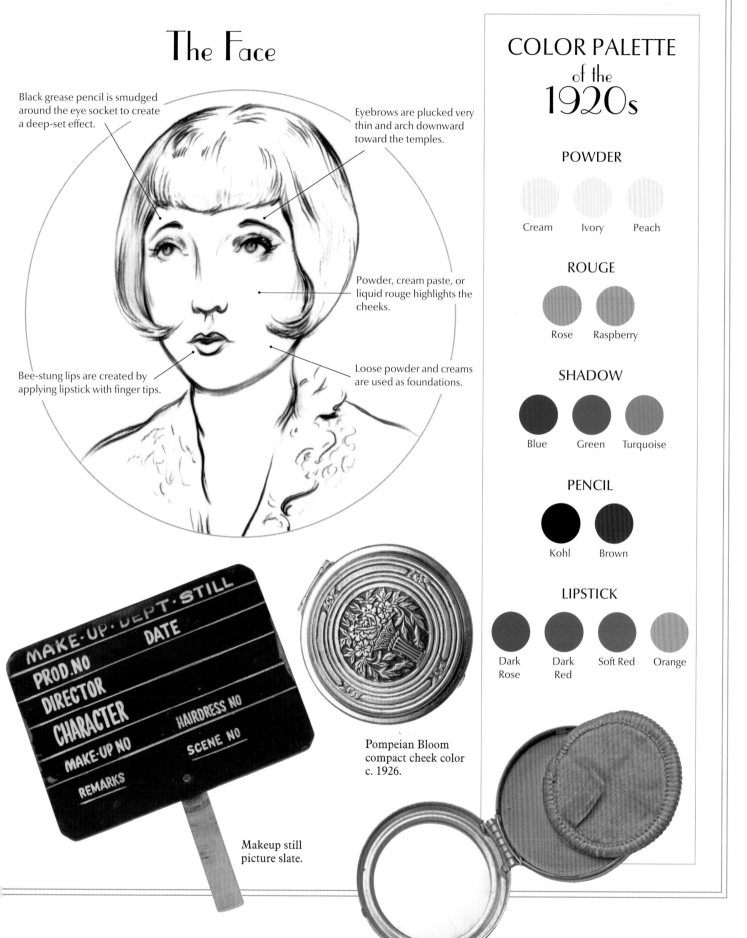

Black grease pencil is smudged around the eye socket to create a deep-set effect.

Eyebrows are plucked very thin and arch downward toward the temples.

Powder, cream paste, or liquid rouge highlights the cheeks.

Bee-stung lips are created by applying lipstick with finger tips.

Loose powder and creams are used as foundations.

Makeup still picture slate.

Pompeian Bloom compact cheek color c. 1926.

COLOR PALETTE
of the
1920s

POWDER

Cream   Ivory   Peach

ROUGE

Rose   Raspberry

SHADOW

Blue   Green   Turquoise

PENCIL

Kohl   Brown

LIPSTICK

Dark Rose   Dark Red   Soft Red   Orange

MAKE·UP·DEPT·STILL
DATE
PROD.NO
DIRECTOR
CHARACTER
HAIRDRESS NO
MAKE-UP NO
SCENE NO
REMARKS

The 1920s Face
A Creation of the Cinema

Eyebrows are black with a downward slope, plucked thin, and filled in with a black grease pencil. Castor or vegetable oil is applied for shine.

Eyes are dusted with dark shadows in green or lampblack.

Lips are shaped like a red Cupid's bow and drawn with a rounded shape on top. Thick waxy red coloring is applied with fingertips avoiding the corners of the mouth. The color is available in a pot, as a liquid, or in a metal case predominantly in orange, red, or dark rose.

Cream and ivory tinted powder and rice powder is applied on top of vanishing cream.

Rose and raspberry rouge in cream or powder paper is applied as a blended circle on each cheek.

Rouge is applied before powder on the lower apples of cheeks in cream paste. Powder is applied on top to soften the look.

Powder rouge is applied after a first coat of powder, followed by a second coat.

Black grease stick eyeliner and wax beads are used on eyelashes.

Facial cream is applied under powder to create a foundation.

Mascara is created from a cake of lampblack powder.

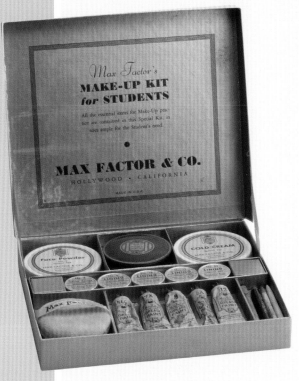

Max Factor student makeup kit for men, c. 1920.

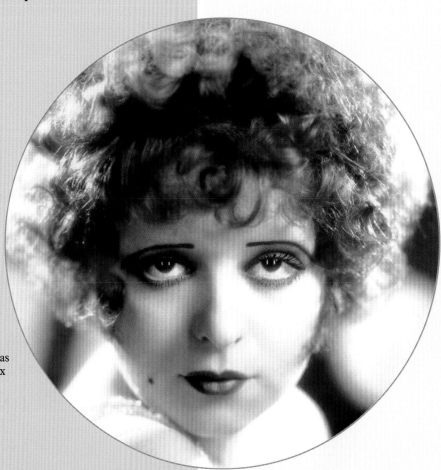

Clara Bow, American silent film star and Roaring '20s sex symbol, photo c. 1920s. Bow was known as the "IT" girl in Hollywood. "IT" was a euphamism for sex appeal.

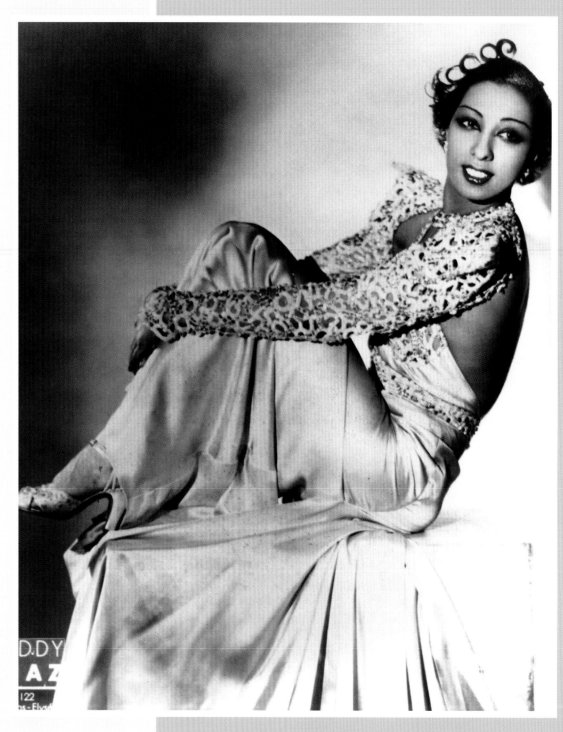

Josephine Baker, first African American entertainer to star in a major motion picture, photo c. 1930. Baker enjoyed her greatest popularity in France, but returned to the USA as a civil rights activist.

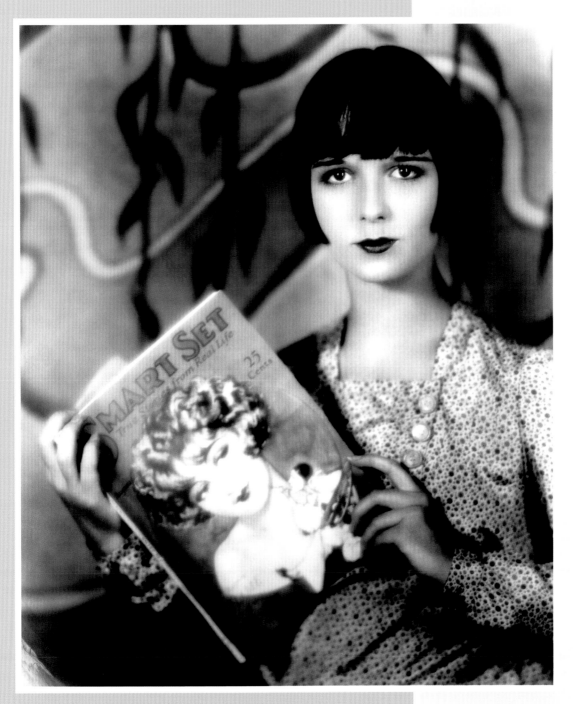

Louise Brooks, American silent film actress known for her bobbed hairdo, photo c. 1920s.

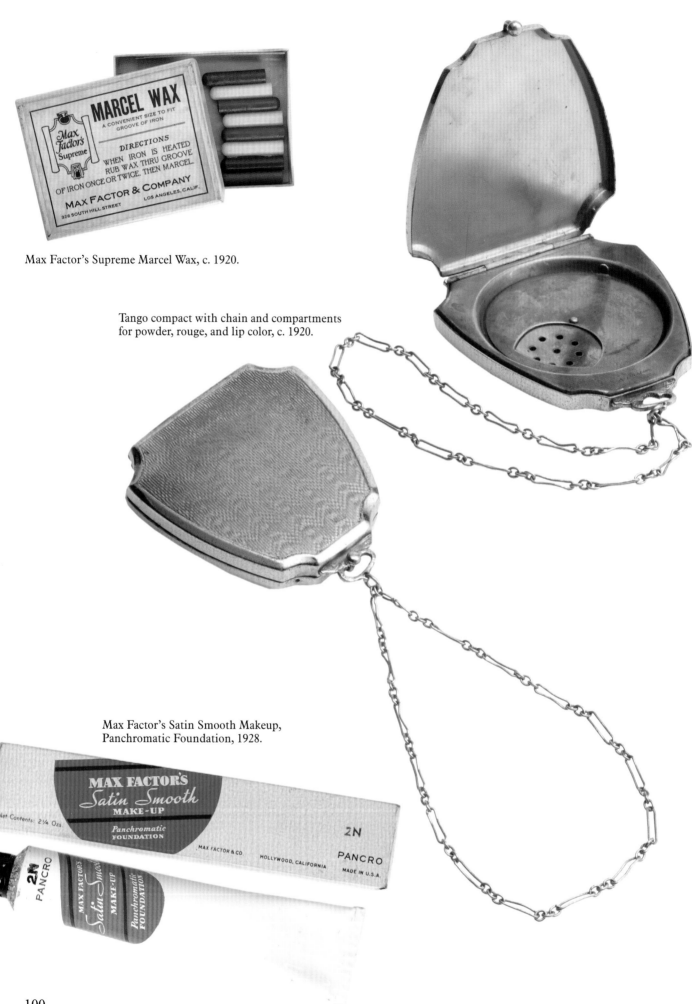

Max Factor's Supreme Marcel Wax, c. 1920.

Tango compact with chain and compartments
for powder, rouge, and lip color, c. 1920.

Max Factor's Satin Smooth Makeup,
Panchromatic Foundation, 1928.

Foundation

A loose powder slightly lighter than one's natural skin tone is used as a primary foundation. Powder is applied with a powder puff over a thin layer of moisturizing cream. The cream provides a moist base for the powder and creates an artificial doll-like complexion.

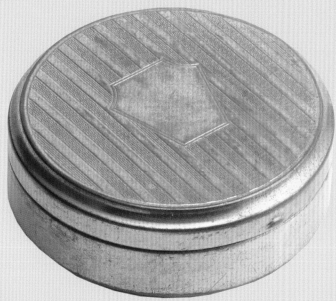

Double decker metal compact for rouge and powder, c. 1920s.

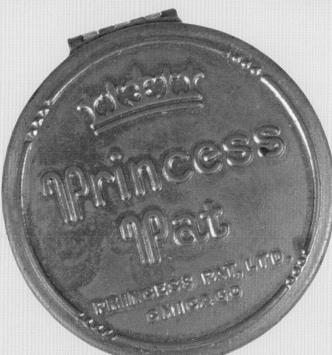

Blush

A powder, cream paste, or liquid rouge is used to highlight the cheeks. The liquid and cream colors are applied to the apples of the cheeks before using the powder foundation.

The powder rouge is applied after the loose powder foundation and is softened by a second application of light powder.

For daytime, rouge is applied to the apples of the cheeks and blended well.

For evening, a circle of rouge is used and blended only at the edges, which leaves a stronger color in the center.

Princess Pat rouge, brass container with mirror on inside of top lid, c. 1920s.

Eyes

Eyebrows are plucked very thin and arched downward toward the temples.

They are enhanced and delineated with a black or brown grease pencil to form an extended curve.

Eyes are elongated with a black grease pencil applied around the eye socket and smudged to create a deep-set effect.

During the day, the eyelids are glossed with lanolin or left bare. Drops of deadly belladonna nightshade, a perennial herb, are used to add sparkle to the whites of the eye.

For night, shadow color is applied to the lid in bright emerald or blue. The lashes are coated with a melted colored wax, similar to a black crayon, which is beaded at the ends of the lashes.

In the mid-'20s, cream mascara made with tinted Vaseline becomes available, which gives lashes a more natural appearance.

Lips

Max Factor creates the bee-stung lips of the era by applying the lipstick on his clients with his fingers. Two prints of his index finger are added to the upper lip, and one print is added across the bottom.

The width of the lips is purposely minimized to create a round pout. The lipstick is also applied with a brush to create the mounded shape, avoiding the corners of the mouth.

Nails

Nails, previously only colored with tinted waxes, are varnished in the center of the nail, leaving the top tip and bottom moon bare. Called the "moon manicure," it is popularized in France.

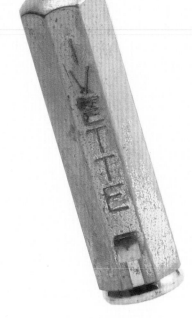

Ivette brand lipstick, brass case with pull-up mechanism, c. 1920.

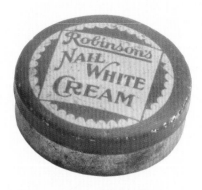

Robinson's brand Nail White Cream, round painted tin, c. 1920s.

Moon manicure.

Historical TIMELINE

A.D. 1930 to A.D. 1938

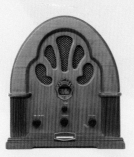

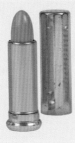

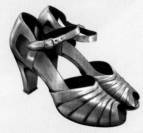

1931
Lady Esther brand promotes cheaper cosmetics with radio advertising.

1936
Max Factor opens his first salon in London. He creates a wide variety of lipstick and powder shades including his famous Pan-Cake makeup. His shiny finish lipstick becomes popular, which leads to the production of other versions by Lancome.

1938
Toenail painting becomes popular with the creation of open-toed evening sandals. Seven shades are available in red tones and black.

1930
The French company Bourjois introduces the perfume Evening in Paris on a radio commercial.

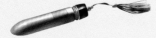

1932
Cosmetics production and distribution improves. Products are easily available in chemist shops as well as department stores. Office girls spend much of their salaries on cosmetics.

1937
Douglas Collins establishes the Goya brand of small bottle perfume. It is sold inexpensively to working women.

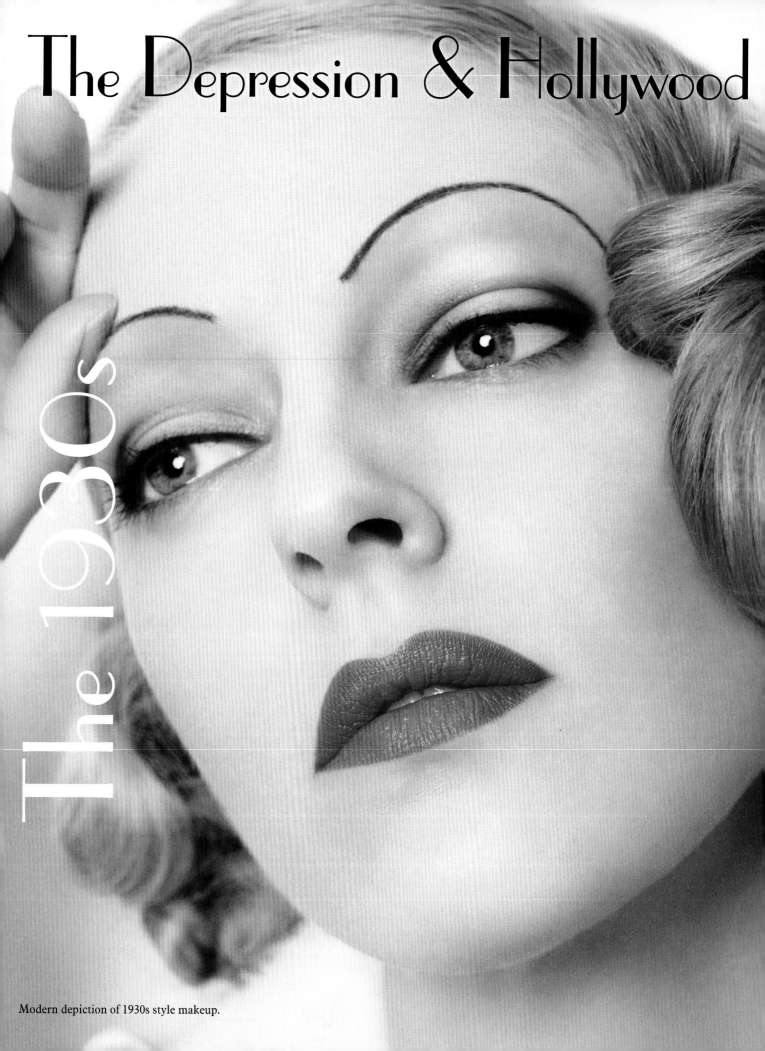

The Depression & Hollywood

The 1930s

Modern depiction of 1930s style makeup.

The Wall Street crash of 1929 made the divide between the rich and the poor wider than ever. Untold numbers of Americans went hungry during more than a decade of joblessness. Women returned to home life and left behind the excesses of the carefree '20s until Hitler's rise in Germany and the eventual outbreak of World War II.

Cosmetics became popular with young women during this time as they gained confidence and independence created by the changing social climate. It was essential to apply a full face of makeup before leaving the house. Beauty routines were introduced by manufacturers that sold complete sets of products. Elizabeth Arden brought about the principle of Color Harmony that matched colors of shadow and rouge to one's wardrobe. Women saw themselves as modern and sophisticated, and looked to cosmetics to help enhance an image of modern beauty. This ideal was heightened and glamorized by the starlets of Hollywood's silver screen. Greta Garbo was considered a screen goddess who exuded sexuality and class.

Escapism was promoted by the movies of the day, which showcased exotic locations, singing, dancing, and formulaic happy endings. This form of mass entertainment provided the optimism needed for a price most could afford. Musicals like *42nd Street* and the comedies of the Marx Brothers were very popular. Fashion among the wealthy imitated what was seen in the movies and was evident in the display of status symbol clothing and accessories. Broad shoulder coats with fox fur and Cartier jewelry were the epitome of style.

Max Factor received much press coverage for the invention of his Pan-Cake makeup, which was widely endorsed by his celebrity clients. He also received attention for two gimmick machines, the "beauty calibrator" and the "kissing machine."

Fashion trends of the decade were influenced by the movies. Women wanted the clothing of the stars, but most could only afford fashions that were more practical for everyday wear. The cloche hat was the preferred shape, and clothing highlighted the female form with a closer fit and feminine drape. Biased cuts provided fluid movement to the garments. Participation in sports for exercise and well-being brought on less constricting fashions suited for fun and relaxation. Again, an element of status and social prestige shaped culture: skiing and tennis in particular were considered elite pastimes. Trousers, backless tops, and shorts were soon popular with active women who wanted to maintain their figures and enjoy the outdoors. By the end of the '30s, chignons and snoods were popular fashion trends.

Hairstyles became softer and more curled. The hair was worn longer, with soft waves and curls, which made the style more sculptured and sensual. Blond hair dominated the decade.

With experimentation and the use of bright and unusual color combinations, colors were more daring. Black nail polish, bright blue and green eye shadows, and orange lips were considered chic.

Decade Highlights

- Elizabeth Arden's salons are so well known that her name becomes the generic term for "beauty salon."
- Ambre Solaire promotes its tanning oil as the ultimate in bronzing care.
- The face with perfectly proportioned bone structure is in fashion.
- Douglas Collins starts Goya perfumes in 1937. He later produces perfumes of good quality in small handbag sizes, which are affordable to the middle-income market.
- Many elaborate movie musicals are produced, such as the surreal, and highly sentimental, *Wizard of Oz* from 1939, which provides a welcome escape from the troubles of reality.
- *Gone with the Wind* is the first motion picture in Technicolor. It brings the development of Pan-Cake makeup by Max Factor, which creates more realistic skin tones and longer lasting coverage for actors in this new brightly colored medium.
- The Preview Combination Set by Germaine Monteil contains cleansing cream, day cream, night cream, powder, and lipstick. This is the first set offered to women as a complete beauty kit.
- Designer cosmetic packaging is introduced with patterns by Lalique for Coty. Yardley perfume bottles are inspired by the Art Nouveau florals of Alphonse Mucha and elegant boxes of Lanvin.
- Tangerine orange scent is popularized by the perfume Californian Poppy. Heavy orange blossoms are rubbed onto clothing and are used as home accents, bringing about the popularity of orange-hued cosmetics.

- Sexuality in films causes musky, sophisticated scents to become more desirable. Light lavender toilette waters are no longer popular and fall out of use.
- Cosmetic availability soars with the opening of Woolworths and other discount chain stores. Advertising is aimed at factory working girls or domestics who have the power to purchase these items for the first time.
- The Allied Forces enter World War II in 1939.
- War rationing efforts make cosmetics hard to find due to limitations on raw materials for manufacturing. Women resort to making creams at home from old formulas. They purchase products on the black market and stockpile products to outlast the war.
- Quality and purity are attributes associated with higher priced items such as Yardley, Elizabeth Arden, Helena Rubinstein, and other French manufacturers. Increased education for shoppers means an awareness of quality, which was missing in the market throughout earlier periods.
- The concentration of industries brings many manufacturers to produce their own brand of products as well as a multitude of smaller private label brands.
- The introduction of color motion pictures makes a huge impact on cosmetic sales. Women imitate the shape of the lips or eyebrows and the exact cosmetic colors seen on actresses.
- Cutex develops a line of nail polishes with matching lip colors.
- "In Hollywood, the lipstick and eyebrow pencil is more powerful than the pen." Perc Westmore, 1931.
- "Beauty is not a gift, it is a habit." Germaine Monteil, 1935.

The Face

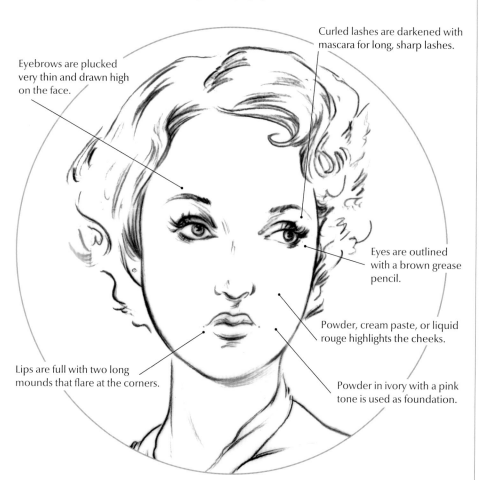

Eyebrows are plucked very thin and drawn high on the face.

Curled lashes are darkened with mascara for long, sharp lashes.

Eyes are outlined with a brown grease pencil.

Powder, cream paste, or liquid rouge highlights the cheeks.

Powder in ivory with a pink tone is used as foundation.

Lips are full with two long mounds that flare at the corners.

COLOR PALETTE
of the
1930s

POWDER

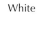

Gardenia Complexion   White

Ivory   Tea Rose   Mauve   Green

ROUGE

Light Pink   Raspberry   Yellow Red   Purple Red

SHADOW

Blue   Green

Purple   Brown   Warm Brown

PENCIL

Brown

LIPSTICK

Light Rose   Raspberry

Chinese Red   Bright Red   Orange

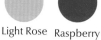

Vanity case in gold metal with compartments for lipstick, powder, a comb, cigarettes, and matches, c. early 1930s.

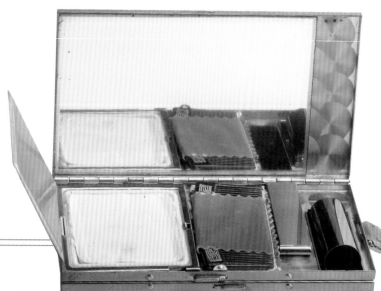

The 1930s Face
The Acceptance of Maquillage

Eyebrows are plucked super thin or are shaved off completely. The new brow is drawn as a thin line that arches down toward the temples. Olive oil or petroleum jelly is applied on the brow for a shiny finish.

For daytime, the eyelids are glossed with a coat of petroleum jelly. Lashes are coated with mascara. For evening, shimmer shadow is used on the upper lid with a dark shadow blended on the crease of the lid to create deep-set eyes. Cream shadow in many bold colors is popular.

As the eyes are kept more natural, kohl liner loses popularity. Dark brown pencil is used to softly line the top and bottom lids without joining the lines on the outside corners of the eye.

Lips are painted with a brush to create a longbow effect for the top lip and a smaller bottom lip. This style is called the rosebud mouth or the "cruller" for the popular pastry.

White or ivory tinted powder with a touch of pink or rice powder is applied on top of vanishing cream.

During the early '30s, rouge is used sparingly if at all. Later in the decade, light applications of pink and raspberry rouge in cream, paste, or liquid are applied high on the cheekbone. Rouge on the upper cheek in cream paste is used before powder, with more powder on top to soften the color. An extra touch of rouge high on the cheeks is used to accentuate the eyes. Powder rouge is applied after the first coat of light powder, followed by a second coat of powder to soften the color to a hint of pink.

Brown or black mascara is used. Henna is commonly worn to darken the eyebrows and eyelashes. Mascara is applied to darken and separate the lashes, not to thicken them. False lashes on the outer corners are used to create a heavy lid effect.

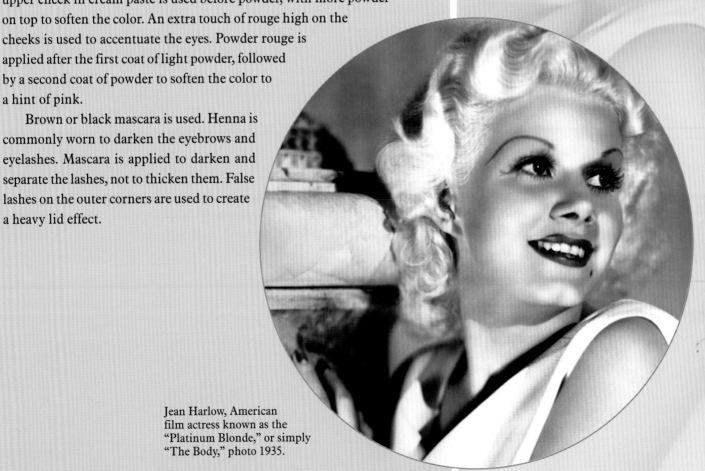

Jean Harlow, American film actress known as the "Platinum Blonde," or simply "The Body," photo 1935.

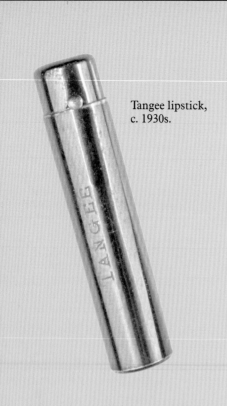

Tangee lipstick,
c. 1930s.

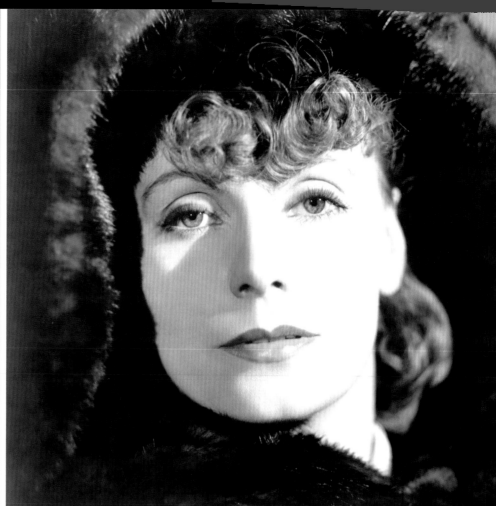

Greta Garbo, Hollywood
screen legend, photo c. 1930s.

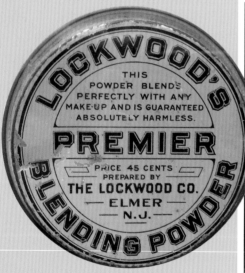

Lockwood's Premier Blending
Powder, blue tin of theatrical makeup
powder, c. 1930s.

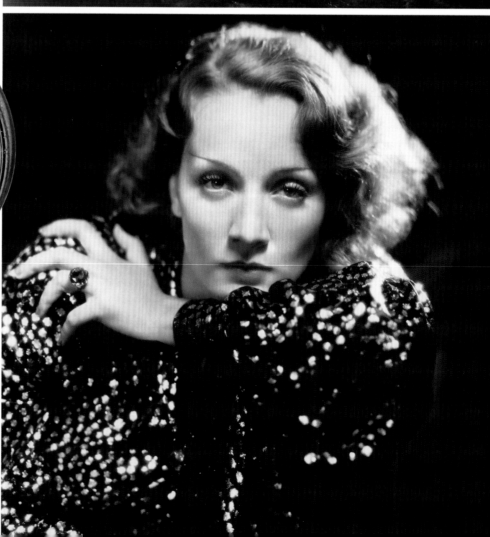

Marlene Dietrich, one of the
highest paid actresses of the
era, photo 1932.

Foundation

A white vanishing cream is used as a base for makeup. Then powder in ivory with a pink tone is used to create a foundation. Later in the decade, powder colors are darker to accommodate tanned skin. Pan-Cake makeup is used in the later part of the decade.

Plough's Cleansing Cream, c. 1930.

Blush

Powder, cream paste, or liquid rouge is used to highlight the cheeks. Liquid and cream colors are applied high on the cheeks before using foundation powder. Powder rouge is applied after loose powder foundation and softened by a second application of light powder. For daytime, light rouge is avoided altogether or applied high on the cheeks and blended well. For evening, rouge is placed near the eyes and blended upward to accentuate the eyes.

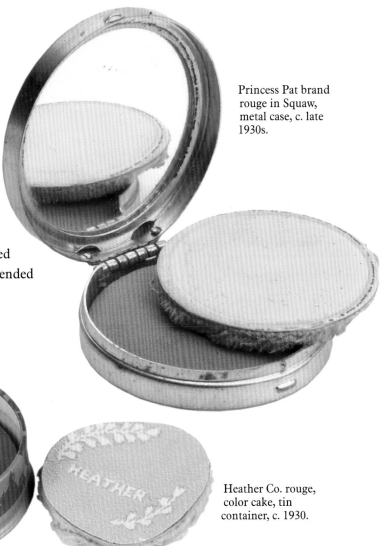

Princess Pat brand rouge in Squaw, metal case, c. late 1930s.

Heather Co. rouge, color cake, tin container, c. 1930.

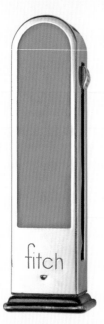

Art Deco style lipstick container from Fitch Co. Brass with push-up mechanism. Blue matte enamel and glossy silver.

Eyes

Eyebrows are plucked to be very thin and are drawn high on the face. A long sweeping curve is drawn and extended to the temples. Eyebrows are coated with oil or petroleum jelly to create sheen.

Eyes are outlined with a brown grease pencil. They are deepened with a light shadow applied on the entire lid and a dark shade that delineates the crease. During the day, eyelids are glossed with oil or left bare. Curled lashes are darkened with mascara to create long, sharp lashes. During the late '30s, shadow colors include blues, greens, and mauves, with silver and gold added to the lid for eveningwear. Lashes are coated with mascara sold in cake form and activated with water to create a paste or petroleum-based cream.

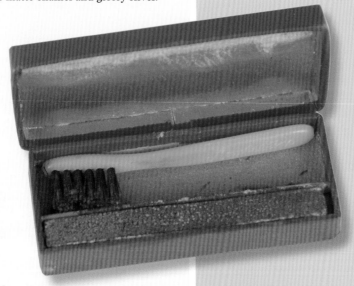

Maybelline mascara, 1932.

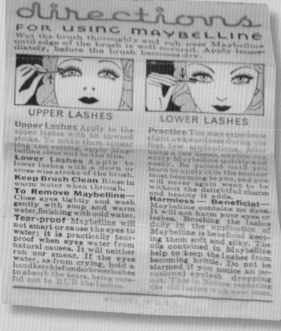

Art Deco Clairol coffin style cake mascara, c. 1930s.

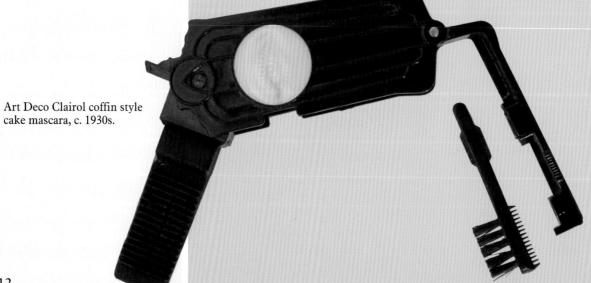

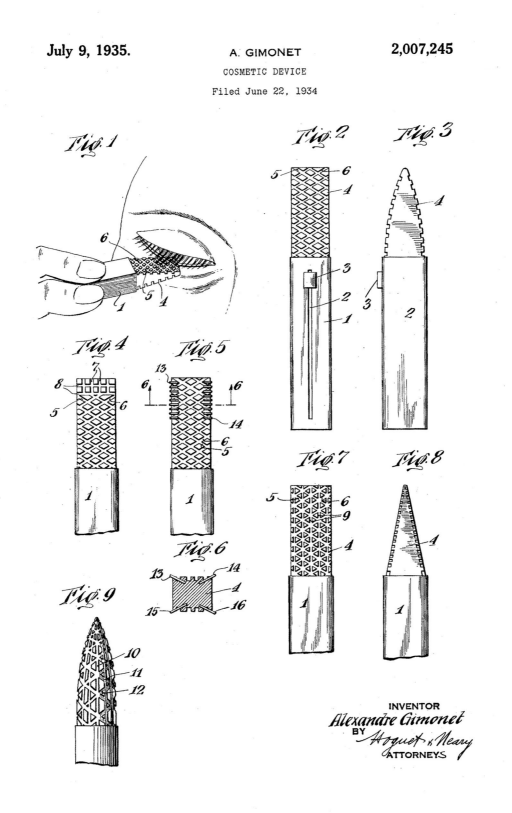

July 9, 1935.　　　　A. GIMONET　　　　2,007,245

COSMETIC DEVICE

Filed June 22, 1934

Fig. 1

Fig. 2

Fig. 3

Fig. 4

Fig. 5

Fig. 6

Fig. 7

Fig. 8

Fig. 9

INVENTOR
Alexandre Gimonet
BY
Hoquet & Neary
ATTORNEYS

Cosmetic Device patent no. 2,007,245 for mascara. A. Gimonet, 1934.

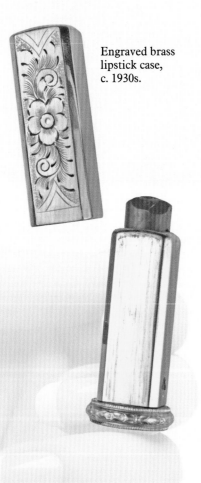

Lips

Lips are full. The top lip is slightly overdrawn and shaped into two long mounds that flare at the corners. Lipstick is used from a tube or with a brush for a more precise application. The pasty nature of lipstick requires the color to be blotted after application.

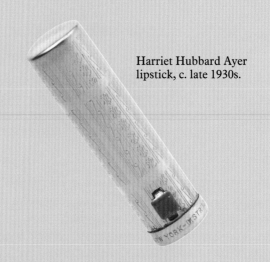

Harriet Hubbard Ayer lipstick, c. late 1930s.

Kissproof Midget lipstick, c. late 1930s.

Engraved brass lipstick case, c. 1930s.

Nails

Nails are varnished in the center of each nail. The top tip and bottom moon are left bare. Earlier in the decade, color choices include light rose, pink, and cream. The year 1932 brings a short-lived trend of painting fingernails black. The end of the decade brings on an expansion of shades available that include red, coral, green, gray, blue, gold, and silver.

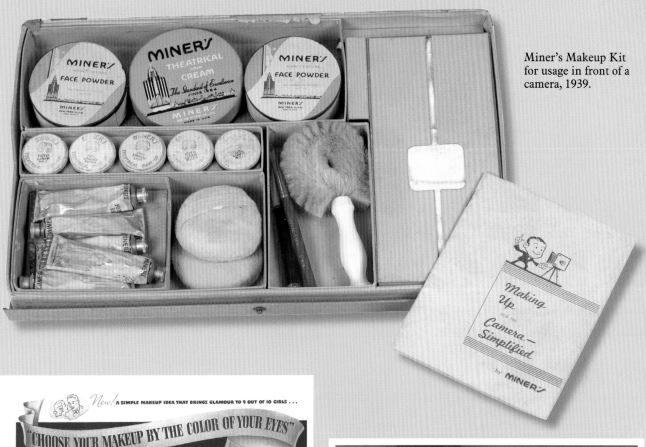

Miner's Makeup Kit for usage in front of a camera, 1939.

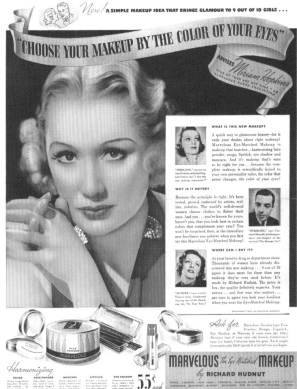

Marvelous Makeup by Richard Hudnut products advertisement, 1937.

Irresistible perfume and beauty aids advertisement, 1935.

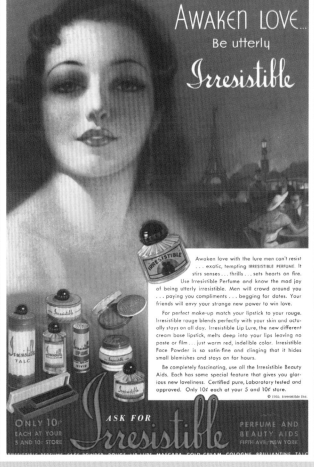

Historical TIMELINE
A.D. 1940 to A.D. 1966

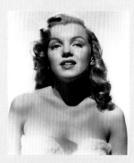

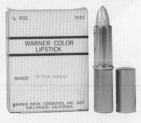

1945
The end of the war marks a return to more feminine styles of clothing and Dior's New Look collection. The industry focuses on novel packaging and a larger array of makeup colors.

1950
The film industry popularizes the blond bombshell Marilyn Monroe and her innocent, spunky, all-American sex appeal. She spurs the sale of bleaching products and even more colors of cosmetics.

1955
Dark red lipstick is replaced with pale tints designed to enhance the summer tanned look. Liquid foundation is introduced.

1946
Americans spend 30 million dollars on cosmetics.

1940
World War II shortages put limitations on the production of cosmetics, which leads to rationing and a black market for lipstick.

Early Technicolor films like *Gone with the Wind*, released January 17, 1940, proved difficult for the makeup artists, especially in this seminal film, which required several actors to age significantly as the story unfolded.

1952
Makeup companies begin creating deeper shades of powder to keep in tune with an increasingly popular suntanned complexion.

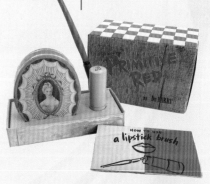

DuBarry Primitive Red Set, contains Primitive Red lipstick, lipstick brush, and 30-day supply of powder, sold for $1.50, c. 1946.

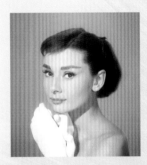

1960
Audrey Hepburn and her continental look make liquid eyeliner popular. The eyes are the most dominant feature of the face, elongated and darkened with the eyeliner.

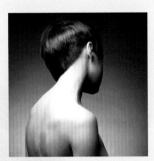

1963
Vidal Sassoon creates sculptural, geometric hair styles and the razor cut hairstyle.

Mary Kay Ash establishes Mary Kay Cosmetics and sells beauty and femininity with home parties and pink Cadillacs.

1966
Mary Quant extends her fashion line to include a cosmetics line.

MARY KAY

1957
Chanel returns to the market after World War II with her cardigan jacket suit and introduces the famous quilted-leather handbag.

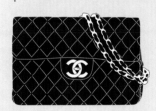

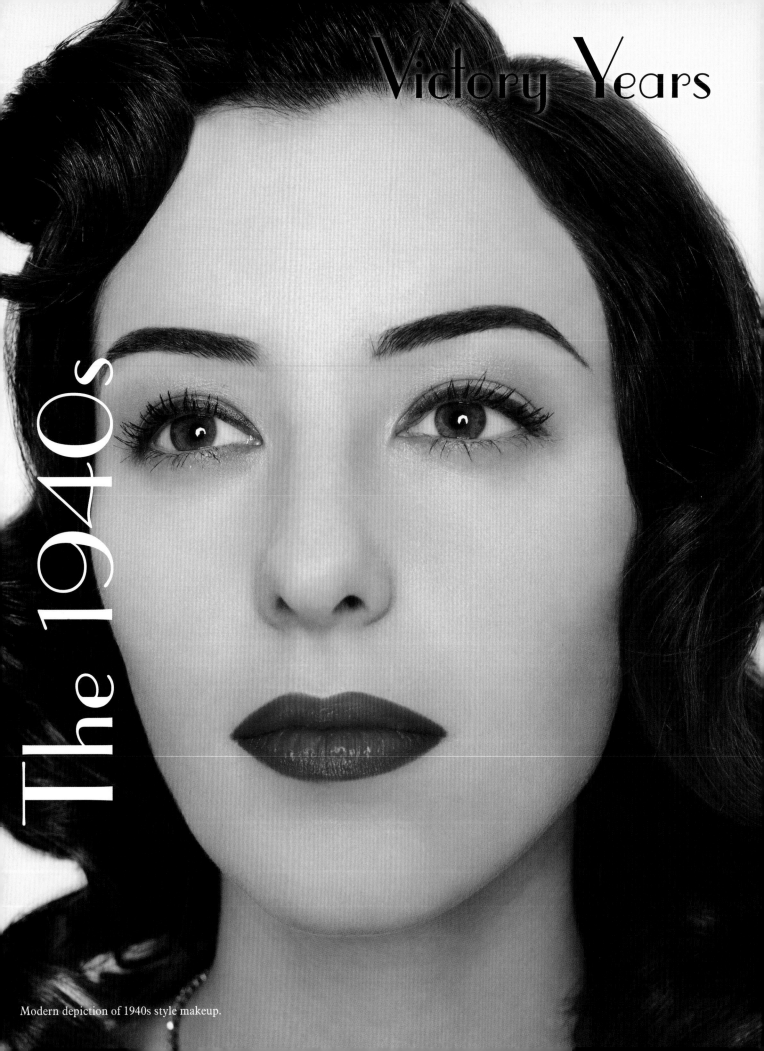

Victory Years

The 1940s

Modern depiction of 1940s style makeup.

The 1940s were an era filled with patriotism, optimism, romance, and glamour. The world was once again at war, and in an effort to boost morale at home and abroad, women were encouraged to look their best while making tremendous personal sacrifices. As with all manufacturing, makeup production was hampered because of shortages in oil, animal fat, and alcohol. Product quality suffered, textures turned dry and flaky, and color choices dwindled.

Hollywood found a way to provide entertainment and reassurance by portraying sultry women and exotic locales in their films. The movies continued to influence cosmetic trends. Products hit the market and were heavily advertised by stars such as Bette Davis, Joan Crawford, Barbara Stanwyck, Vivien Leigh, Ginger Rogers, and Myrna Loy. Women used Pan-Stik and Pan-Cake foundations in the hopes of achieving the smooth, flawless complexions of Hollywood's most famous starlets.

The standard face of the '40s was made up simply with arched penciled brows, powder, and large red lips. The use of bright red lipstick had such an impact on morale for women during World War II that it has become forever linked to improving confidence and as a symbol of victory.

A more natural look with a healthy rosy complexion was desirable throughout the '40s. Hair was longer and styled with elaborate rolls. Wavy locks covered one eye. Topknots and hair kerchiefs in the "Rosie the Riveter" style were worn as a practical way of dealing with medium length hair while at work. The hair was pushed up, formed a crown of curls, and was usually wrapped in a turban scarf.

Women in Britain were still wearing the Marcel wave, and shorter permed styles were popular for women in service uniforms. After the war, the Joan of Arc style made popular by Ingrid Bergman, began the gamine style of the '50s. Hairpieces were often used to forego visits to the hairdresser. False braids, bangs, and combs with curls were used to create elegant evening styles.

Trade restrictions, lack of supplies, and overall costs limited even the most everyday necessities during the war years. Metal used in jewelry, cosmetic cases, and clothing fasteners, was strictly to be used in making supplies for the war effort. Silk, once coveted in fashion, was restricted for the manufacturing of military parachutes. Factories were converted into war supply production facilities where women labored to make everything from ammunition to aircraft. They wore the tough uniforms worn by men. Jeans and t-shirts became acceptable casual attire amongst women.

Besides working in the factories, women became part of the war effort after Congress passed legislation that created the Women's Army Corps, the Women's Reserves of the Navy, and the Coast Guard Women's Reserves. Females who served in the corps did so as pilot instructors, airplane mechanics, clerical workers, and even airplane pilots.

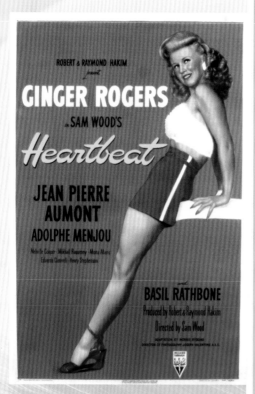

Poster for the film *Heartbeat*, starring Ginger Rogers, 1946.

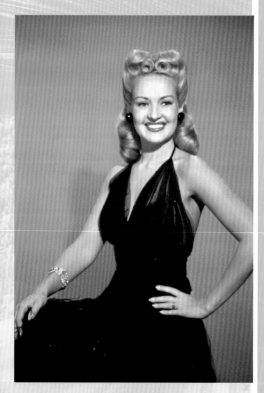

Betty Grable in the Film *Springtime in the Rockies*, 1942.

Clothing designers focused on making attire for the working woman, but fabric shortages made the styles stiff and narrow. The skirt was shorter, and the waist was clearly marked using every trick to save fabric. Fashion trends included trousers with narrow hips and jackets with wide shoulders. Hats and gloves were a must to provide some femininity to the plain suit styles. For casual wear, trousers and platform shoes accompanied the more active working lifestyle. The slightly mannish Katharine Hepburn wore her tailored trousers with aristocratic American optimism in a number of films.

Costume jewelry was a popular fashion accessory in America, and designer pieces by Miriam Haskell became prized possessions. Underwear was scarce, so many women began tailoring their own. Tight satin underwear with stitching became the standard. It was pulled up and rolled onto the body because it did not contain zippers due to the rationing of metal. The rubber corset was introduced, but proved to be unpopular.

During the war, Britain saw a change in the attitude of the elite social class. People were brought together in the spirit of patriotism. The soldier's uniform became the acceptable fashion for everyone. Rationing was even more severe. Women's publications advised them to make do with what they had and mend old clothing, curtains, and sheets.

France was divided between those who collaborated with the Nazis and those who supported the resistance forces. Women wore whatever met the needs of their mission, blending in by wearing civilian or peasant clothing, or wearing overtly sexy clothing to attract the attention of the German soldiers. Some women used clothing as a dangerous display of their opposition and adopted very tall colorful hats and short skirts.

After the war, technological developments flooded the market with new products, which included fluid eyeliner, cake liner, eye shadow sticks, waterproof cream mascara, makeup removers, and eyelash curlers. Eyeliner became an important cosmetic with the return of the darker doe-eyed look. Eyeliner pencil, eye shadow and mascara were must-have products for every beauty-conscious female.

The development of television spurred the creation of many niche brands as specialized products advertised in this new medium. Tangee lipstick ads proclaimed that lipstick symbolized "the precious right of women to be feminine and lovely—under any circumstance."

Decade Highlights

- Dior's New Look collection debuts in 1947 and gives women a sense of femininity, elegance, and a new approach to dressing.
- The Cannes Film Festival is inaugurated in 1947.
- Pan-Stik makeup by Max Factor is sold in Europe.
- Beauty patches are re-introduced to accompany the "painted look."
- The ballet shoe, made by Capezio, becomes fashionable.
- Dior creates his perfume company with the launch of Miss Dior.
- The bras of the era are conical in shape, resembling missiles with circular stitching.
- Leg makeup becomes popular as a replacement for stockings not available during the war. In Britain, girls use tea or brown food dye to achieve a natural tanned leg.
- Claire McCardell develops American casual wear. Her clothes have a timeless quality, influencing Calvin Klein and Ralph Lauren as well as many other current designers.
- England's Dr. McIndoe's advances in plastic surgery for war injuries, pioneers the science of skin donation and reconstruction surgeries.
- After the war, an abundance of nylon makes stockings inexpensive and affordable to all.
- Frederick's of Hollywood introduces edible underwear and musical underpants. These outrageous firsts define the brand as a provider of provocative undergarments.
- Coco Chanel introduces her range of lipsticks.
- Lancaster, named after the Lancaster bomber, introduces Serum Tissulaire and Crème Embryonnaire, predecessors to today's beauty creams.
- After 1945, women wore their hair in "Victory Rolls."
- Betty Grable is the most popular pin-up girl and has her legs insured for one million dollars.
- Lena Horne is the first black performer to have a long-term contract with Hollywood studio MGM, even though this *Stormy Weather* icon often had to pose and pass as Latina to find a meal or a hotel room while on tour in the USA because of Jim Crow laws.

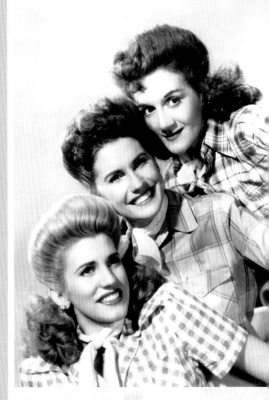

The Andrews Sisters, U.S. vocal group about 1943. From top: LaVerne, Patty, and Maxene.

The Face

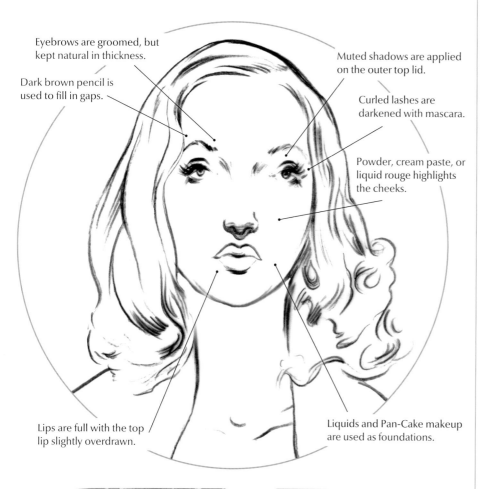

Eyebrows are groomed, but kept natural in thickness.

Dark brown pencil is used to fill in gaps.

Muted shadows are applied on the outer top lid.

Curled lashes are darkened with mascara.

Powder, cream paste, or liquid rouge highlights the cheeks.

Lips are full with the top lip slightly overdrawn.

Liquids and Pan-Cake makeup are used as foundations.

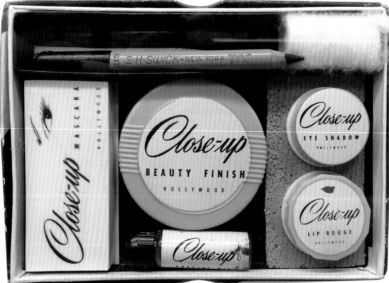

Close-up makeup kit, c. 1940s.

COLOR PALETTE
of the
1940s

LIQUID FOUNDATION

Warm
Skin

POWDER

Ivory   Flesh

ROUGE

Red/   Bright Pink/   Rose
Pink   Fuchsia

SHADOW

Gray   Brown

PENCIL

Dark Brown

LIPSTICK

Pink Red   Orange
Red

Deep   Bright   Cherry
Red   Red   Red

The 1940s Face
The Natural Beauty

Eyebrows are natural in thickness and filled in with brown pencil. Arches are manicured into clean, defined shapes. Stray hairs are tweezed, and the space between the brows is kept clean. Brown pencil is used lightly to enhance the shape of the arch and to darken very fair hair.

For daytime, eyelids are worn with a light shadow. Lashes are coated with mascara. For evening, muted shadow colors are used on the crease and the outer edge of the lid. Liner is rarely used, as the eyes are kept more natural.

Lips are painted to look full with added roundness on the mounds of the top lip. Applied with a brush or from the tube, the top lip is slightly overdrawn, and the color is spread from the center to the outer edges of the lips. Glycerin is used to gloss the lips.

Face powder matches one's skin tone, but still contains pink undertones. A darker liquid foundation is layered with a lighter powder.

Cheeks are kept natural. Rouge is used high on the cheekbones and blended up toward the temples for a subtle rosy glow. It is believed that blending rouge upward would make eyes brighter. Rouge is available in a powder, paste, or liquid.

Mascara was brown or black. It was used to darken the lashes and was applied heavily on the outer corners of the eyes.

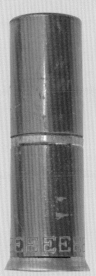

Elizabeth Arden Radiant Peony lipstick, c. 1944.

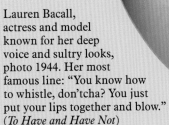

Lauren Bacall, actress and model known for her deep voice and sultry looks, photo 1944. Her most famous line: "You know how to whistle, don'tcha? You just put your lips together and blow." (*To Have and Have Not*)

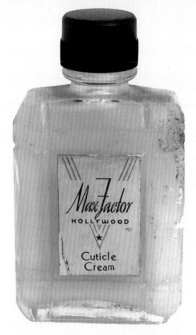

Max Factor Hollywood Cuticle Cream,
c. 1940.

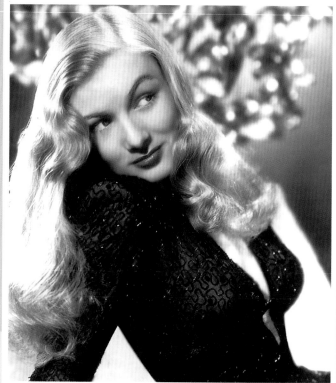

Veronica Lake, American
film actress and pin-up
model, famous for her femme
fatale roles and her hairstyle
that covered one eye, photo
c. 1940s.

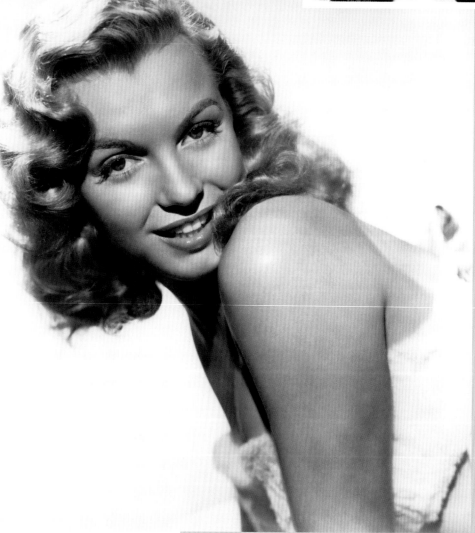

Marilyn Monroe, Hollywood
sex symbol and superstar,
photo 1946—the early,
freshly scrubbed years.

Foundation

Foundations are now available in liquids and Pan-Cake. Creams or liquids are used lightly on the face and neck, and dusted off with a light powder for a matte finish. For lighter applications, the moisturizer, followed with a light powder, is used as a base.

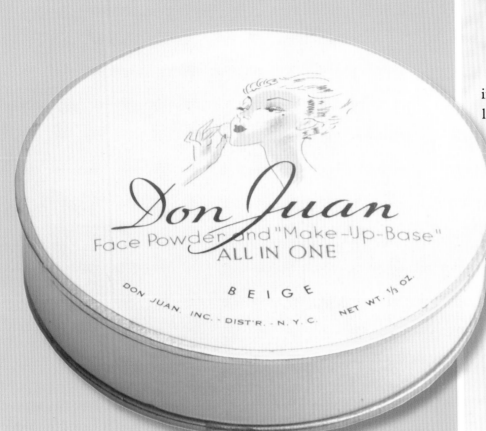

Don Juan Face Powder and Makeup Base in Beige, cardboard case with printed label, c. early 1940s.

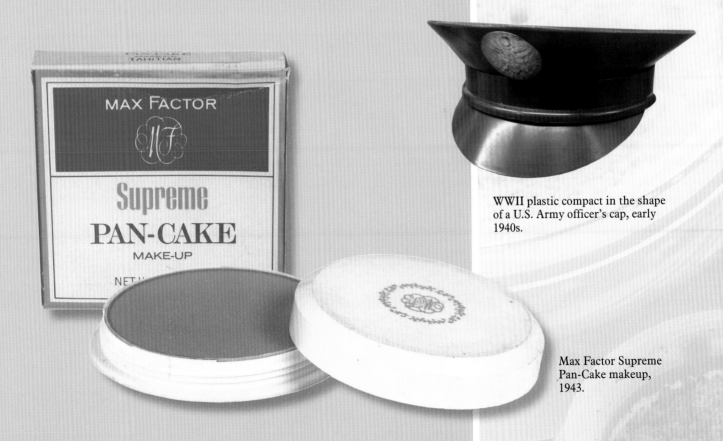

WWII plastic compact in the shape of a U.S. Army officer's cap, early 1940s.

Max Factor Supreme Pan-Cake makeup, 1943.

Blush

Rouge, in the form of powder, cream paste, or liquid, is used to highlight the cheeks. A subtle and natural blushing effect is favored. The color is applied high on the cheeks and blended upward.

Eyes

Eyebrows are kept manicured but fairly natural in thickness. A natural arched curve is preferred. Dark brown pencil is used to fill in gaps or to darken light hairs. Eyelids are kept light. Muted shadows are applied to the outer top lid as the shadow delineated the crease. During the day, the eyelids are left bare. Curled lashes are darkened with mascara applied to the outer corner of the lashes.

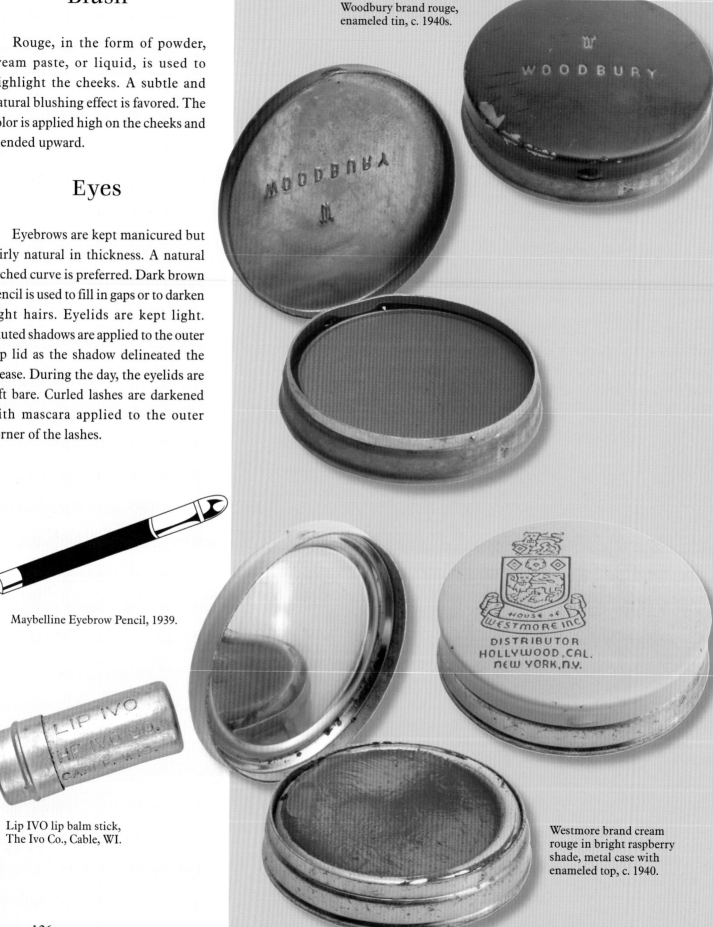

Woodbury brand rouge, enameled tin, c. 1940s.

Maybelline Eyebrow Pencil, 1939.

Lip IVO lip balm stick, The Ivo Co., Cable, WI.

Westmore brand cream rouge in bright raspberry shade, metal case with enameled top, c. 1940.

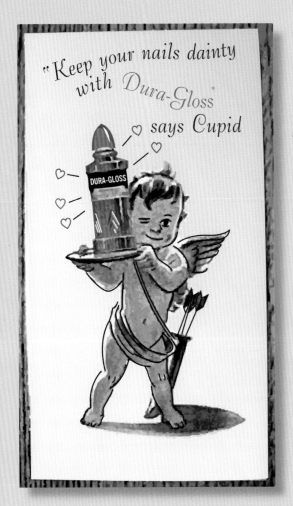

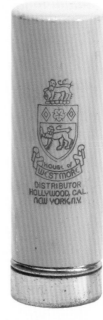

Lips

The top lip is slightly overdrawn, creating a full lip. Lipstick is applied directly from the tube or with a brush for a more detailed application.

Westmore brand mini lipstick, metal enameled tube, c. 1940.

Dura-Gloss nail polish advertisement, c. 1944.

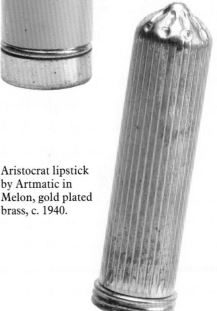

Aristocrat lipstick by Artmatic in Melon, gold plated brass, c. 1940.

Cutex brand Alert nail polish by designer Schiaparelli advertisement, c. 1945.

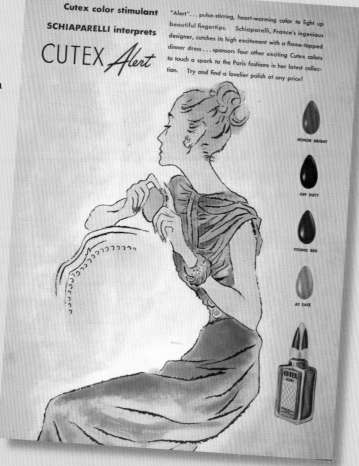

Nails

Nails are varnished except for a thin curve at the top and the bottom moon, which are both free of paint. Nail colors match clothing with colors that include red, green, yellow, black, blue, and plum.

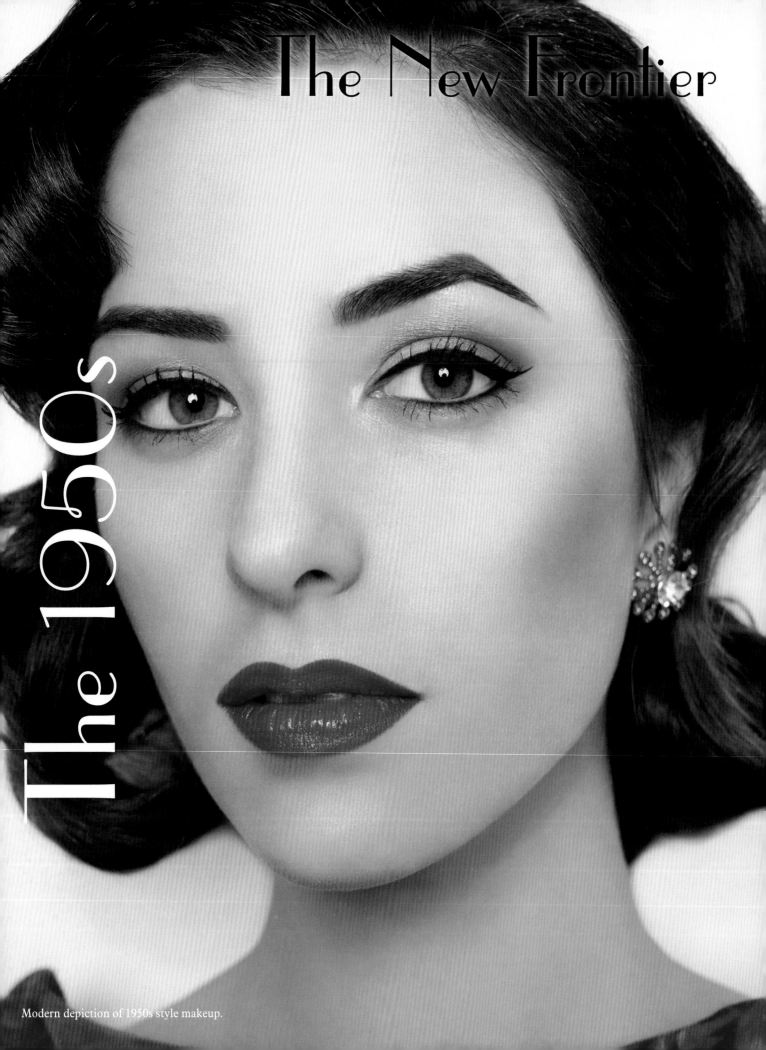

The New Frontier

The 1950s

Modern depiction of 1950s style makeup.

After their brief stint as factory workers during the war, women were once again the matriarchs of the home. They were expected to marry and raise a family while men returned to the role of the breadwinner, reprising American society's most conventional and conformist roles. The Cold War and a national paranoia about communism, led by Senator Joseph McCarthy, enforced conservatism. Fear of nuclear attack from the USSR created a "bunker mentality" at home in the suburbs. But some women challenged this stifling Suburban fantasy and worked outside the home, out of financial need or simple boredom. This new career woman was portrayed as cold and intimidating, and it was assumed that she had not found the right man to marry.

The war's victory brought on prosperity and a new affluent lifestyle for Americans. The advent of credit made even luxury items, i.e. mink coats and Cadillacs, readily available. Success was measured by the collection of possessions as consumerism rose and improved the standard of living. New products were created to meet the demands of this new society. Technology developed by the military during the war created advancements in automation for home appliances, synthetic materials, television, and jet engines. Most advertisements of the period showcased products aimed at housewives who were in charge of their home's upkeep.

Even though American manufacturing was superior, Paris remained the capital of style and fashion. Models began to enjoy the perks only held by high society women, becoming personalities named in the social columns of the time. Grace Kelly represented the face of the ideal woman.

Cosmetic advertisers now used professional models in highly stylized images. As women searched for refinement in their cosmetic products, manufacturers catered to this need by focusing on chic locales, like Paris, or romantic and exciting product names that brought a sense of fantasy to the industry. The eye was a prominent feature. A new Egyptian shape characterized by thicker eyeliner and more defined shadow became a popular look during the era. Wearing makeup was a must for all occasions as women were expected to look good at all times.

Eye shadow, liner, and mascara colors were daring and bold, and heavily applied. Violet, blue, silver, and copper frost were the colors of the day. Modernity meant wearing bright colors with sharp, angular makeup, although lips were painted with neutral shades to promote a pouty, sex-kitten look.

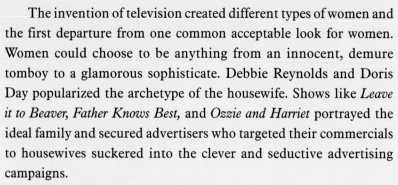

The invention of television created different types of women and the first departure from one common acceptable look for women. Women could choose to be anything from an innocent, demure tomboy to a glamorous sophisticate. Debbie Reynolds and Doris Day popularized the archetype of the housewife. Shows like *Leave it to Beaver, Father Knows Best,* and *Ozzie and Harriet* portrayed the ideal family and secured advertisers who targeted their commercials to housewives suckered into the clever and seductive advertising campaigns.

Estée Lauder's Youth Dew was the first perfume to be marketed to women as a self-purchase. Women were encouraged to buy the perfume on their own instead of waiting for a man to give it to them as a gift.

Teens with money to spend became a force in the marketplace. Young girls began to go against their parents' wishes and established their own styles of dress and makeup, influenced by music—the beginnings of rock n' roll—far more so than movies or books. They wore bright lipstick and eye makeup, tight jeans and sweaters, and danced to the wild sounds of rock n' roll. Audrey Hepburn's pixie cut and gamin look, and Brigitte Bardot's sex-kitten look were the styles favored by young teens.

The fifties showcased many different hairstyle trends. Blonde was considered the ideal hair color. Home dyes and extensive experimentation with hairpieces and accessories were extremely popular. Bobbed hair was a top trend. Later in the decade, the "ratted," or back-combed, bouffant and beehive were worldwide trends that required the use of large rollers and heavy hair sprays. Hairdressers became indispensable to women, as weekly trips to set the hair were the norm. The larger hairstyles curbed the chic wearing of hats, as only the simplest of styles survived into the 1960s.

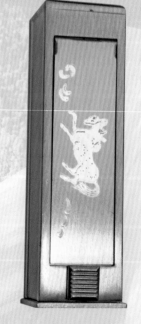

Elgin lipstick holder case with a horse decoration engraved on the flip up mirror. An ingenious purse accessory that simply pulls apart from the bottom to top. The patented mechanism allows the lid to pop open.

Decade Highlights

- The first disposable lipstick case appears. Packaging becomes less adorned and more utilitarian.
- The body shape of a woman changes to a more muscular, curvy figure, with pointed breasts accentuated by circular-stitched bras. The breast becomes the new erogenous zone.
- Howard Hughes invents the cantilevered bra. It becomes a popular choice under strapless dresses.
- Girlie pajamas and Babydolls, worn by teens, are popularized at slumber parties as depicted in B movies and television shows.
- The bikini becomes popular after the French actress Brigitte Bardot wears it in films.
- The middle class aspires to a highly materialistic lifestyle. Activities like cocktail and dinner parties and sports like tennis and golf, previously reserved for the upper class, are now affordable and ever-desirable.
- With the popularization of rock n' roll, Elvis Presley becomes a household name as music becomes part of the new lifestyle.
- New foundations like Touch and Glow and Love Pat bring about a dewy moist look to the face.
- Aziza sells mascara and establishes a niche in the market.
- "Most women lead lives of dullness, of quiet desperation. Cosmetics are a wonderful escape from it—if you play it right." Martin Revson, VP of Revlon, 1952.
- *Playboy* publishes its' first issue in 1953 featuring a nude photograph of the then brunette Marilyn Monroe.

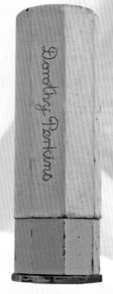

Dorothy Perkins lipstick in "Medium", c. 1950s.

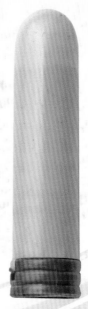

Seduction Paris lipstick, c. 1950s.

The Face

Eyebrows are thicker, darker, and shaped with a prominent arch.

Doe eyes consist of soft, full lashes, black liner, and light shadow.

Natural cream or liquid foundation is used as a makeup base.

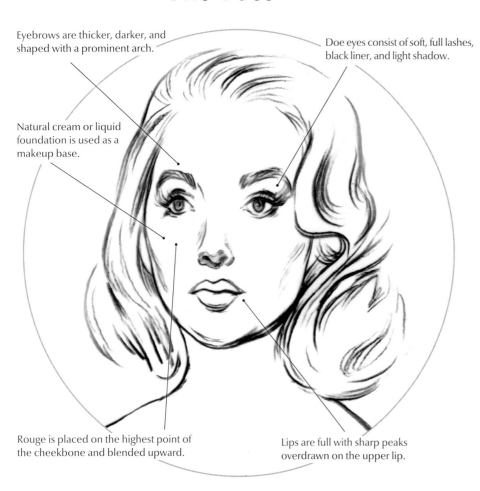

Rouge is placed on the highest point of the cheekbone and blended upward.

Lips are full with sharp peaks overdrawn on the upper lip.

Ingrid Bergman, Swedish actress and international screen star, wholesome yet sultry, photo c. 1950s.

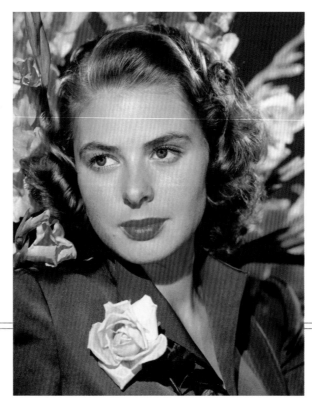

COLOR PALETTE of the 1950s

POWDER

Lotus Lily Green · Flesh · Rachel

ROUGE

Light Pink · Rose

Coral · Peach · Pink/Orange

SHADOW

Light Blue · Turquoise

True Gray · Brown · Sapphire

Gold · Silver

MASCARA

Black · Brown · Blue

LIPSTICK

Deep Red · Fuchsia

Bright Pink · Coral · Pink/Orange

The 1950s Face
Doe-Eyed Makeup

Eyebrows are thick, well shaped and worn with a high arch. The pronounced arch starts in the middle of the brow. Brown or dark black pencil is used to darken and shape the brow regardless of the color of the hair.

Eyes are lengthened with a black pencil to create a doe-eyed effect. Black pencil lines the top lid, and extends the line past the outer corner, arching upward. The lower lid is lined to meet the top line. Shadow is used on the top lid, extending to the outer corner. Younger girls also wear this look with brown and pink shadow as a base.

Defined peaks on the top lip create full lips. The new bow of the lip is done by using different intensities of color, drawing the V-shaped bow with two short lines, filling the rest of the lip from the corners to the bow. Younger girls use pale pink lip color to create a full, pouty lip. The lip pencil is not available, so girls use brown eyebrow pencils to define the lips.

Pearl color foundation is finished with a dusting of flesh-colored powder. Foundation is available in liquid, cream, and pressed powder. The Lotus Lily complexion is achieved with green powder over natural foundation, creating a light finish. Liquid and cream are set with a natural shade powder. Younger girls use a tan base lightly, and avoid the matte look of powder.

Rouge contours the cheeks to define the bones. Color is applied on the cheek bones and blended upward. Younger girls do not use blush and prefer to define only the eyes and lips.

Mascara in black or brown is used only on the upper lashes.

Audrey Hepburn, legendary British actress, Oscar winner, and humanitarian, cherished for her elfin title role in *Sabrina*, photo c. 1950s.

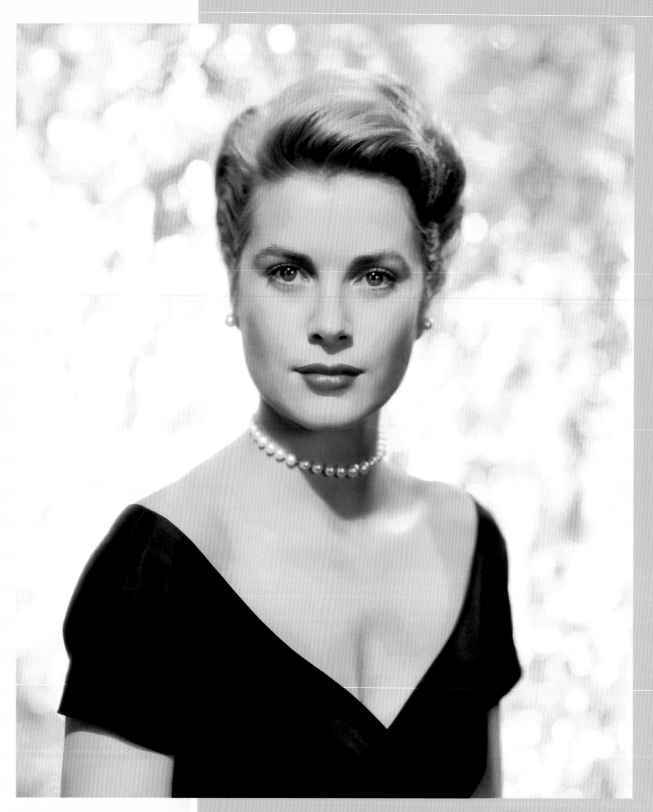

Truly an American royal.
Grace Kelly, glamorous film star and princess of Monaco, photo 1956.

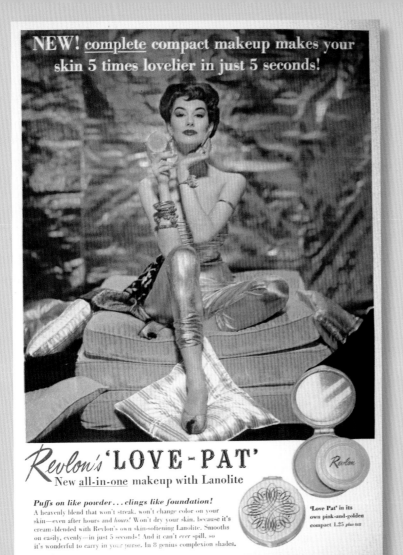

NEW! **complete** compact makeup makes your skin 5 times lovelier in just 5 seconds!

Revlon's 'LOVE-PAT'
New **all-in-one** makeup with Lanolite

Puffs on like powder... clings like foundation!
A heavenly blend that won't streak, won't change color on your skin—even after hours and *hours!* Won't dry your skin, because it's cream-blended with Revlon's own skin-softening Lanolite. Smooths on easily, evenly—in just 5 seconds! And it can't *ever* spill, so it's wonderful to carry in your purse. In 8 genius complexion shades.

'Love Pat' in its own pink-and-golden compact 1.25 *plus tax*

Foundation

A natural cream or liquid foundation is used as a base for makeup. Flesh colored powder or ivory with a pink tone is used to set the foundation. Lighter powder over a darker foundation is also used for effect, and high fashion women tend to choose lighter foundations. Light green powder is used for a brightening effect. The face remains matte, and the prominent use of tinted powder matches the liquid foundation.

Revlon brand Love-Pat foundation compact advertisement, 1954.

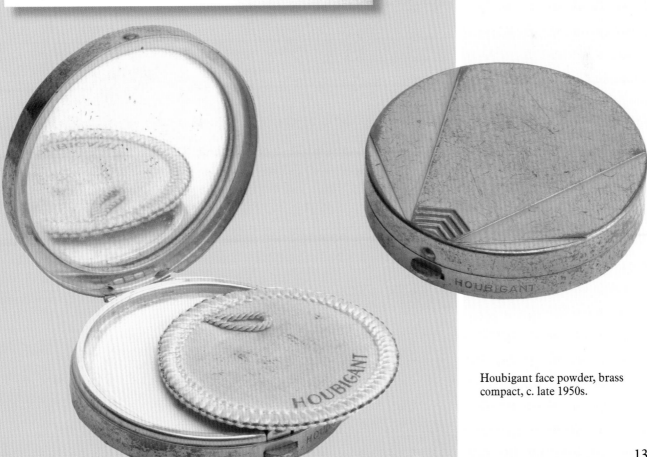

Houbigant face powder, brass compact, c. late 1950s.

Blush

Rouge colors become more muted as peach-colored cheeks become more popular than pink. Rouge is placed on the highest point of the cheekbone and blended up. Powder rouge is preferred with the increase of the use of application brushes instead of puffs.

Eyes

Eyebrows are darkened with a black or brown pencil, thicker, darker, and display a prominent arch. They are groomed to look clean and bold.

The doe-eyed look consists of soft full lashes, black liner, and light shadow. A muted light shadow is used on the entire lid, extending to the eyebrow. A darker shade is used in the crease and blended up toward the temples. From the inner corner of the eye, a line ranging from thin to thick is drawn, and extends out and upward past the outer corner of the eye. Lower lashes are lined, and join the upper line at the outer corner.

The most popular shadow colors are green and gray followed by blue and neutral. Shadow is applied on the lid and extends out to the side.

Cake mascara is still used, but the mascara wand makes thicker lashes possible with less effort. Most women use mascara only on the top lashes. Models and celebrities use false lashes.

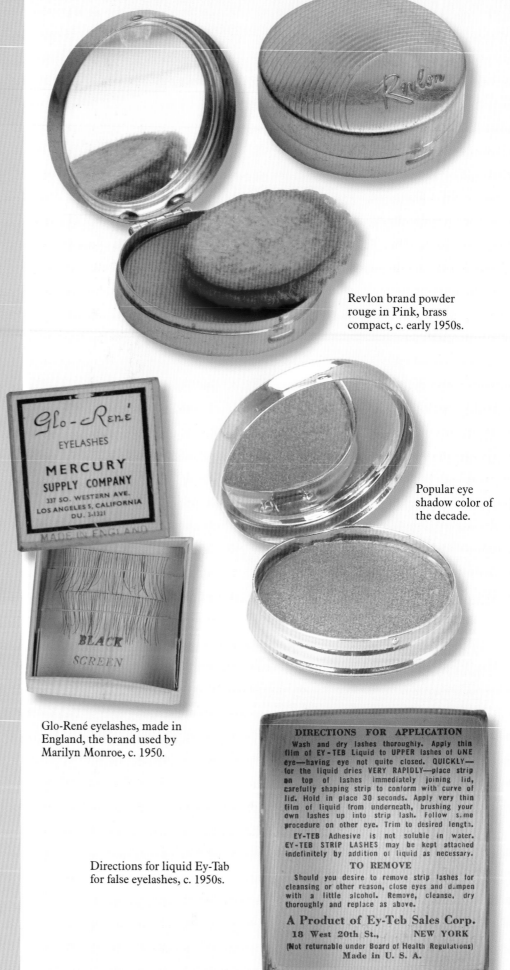

Revlon brand powder rouge in Pink, brass compact, c. early 1950s.

Popular eye shadow color of the decade.

Glo-René eyelashes, made in England, the brand used by Marilyn Monroe, c. 1950.

Directions for liquid Ey-Tab for false eyelashes, c. 1950s.

DIRECTIONS FOR APPLICATION

Wash and dry lashes thoroughly. Apply thin film of EY-TEB Liquid to UPPER lashes of ONE eye—having eye not quite closed. QUICKLY—for the liquid dries VERY RAPIDLY—place strip on top of lashes immediately joining lid, carefully shaping strip to conform with curve of lid. Hold in place 30 seconds. Apply very thin film of liquid from underneath, brushing your own lashes up into strip lash. Follow same procedure on other eye. Trim to desired length.

EY-TEB Adhesive is not soluble in water. EY-TEB STRIP LASHES may be kept attached indefinitely by addition of liquid as necessary.

TO REMOVE

Should you desire to remove strip lashes for cleansing or other reason, close eyes and dampen with a little alcohol. Remove, cleanse, dry thoroughly and replace as above.

A Product of Ey-Teb Sales Corp.

18 West 20th St., NEW YORK

(Not returnable under Board of Health Regulations)

Made in U. S. A.

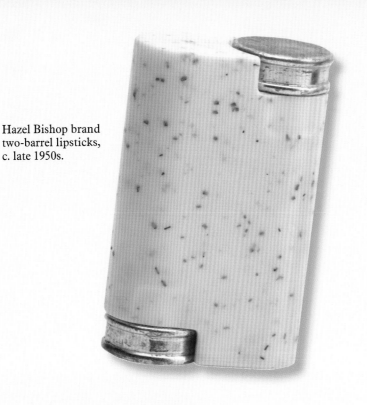

Hazel Bishop brand
two-barrel lipsticks,
c. late 1950s.

Lips

Sharp peaks overdrawn on the
upper lip create full lips. Lipstick is
applied from the tube or with a brush
for a more detailed application. Bright
shades of red are used in the beginning
of the decade and change to paler colors
by the mid-'50s. True red, orange,
and pink colors are used at the end of
the decade. Very pale pink colors are
popular with younger girls.

Nails

Revlon brand
Indelible lipstick,
brass top swivel tube,
c. 1950.

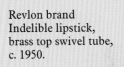

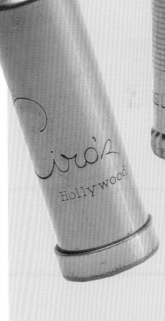

Ciro's
Hollywood
brand lipstick
by Dover in
dark violet
shade, c. late
1950s.

Nails are painted to match the
color of the lipstick. Color is applied to
the entire nail, with color layering and
mixing for different effects.

Cutex brand Midget Manicure Set, c. early 1950s.

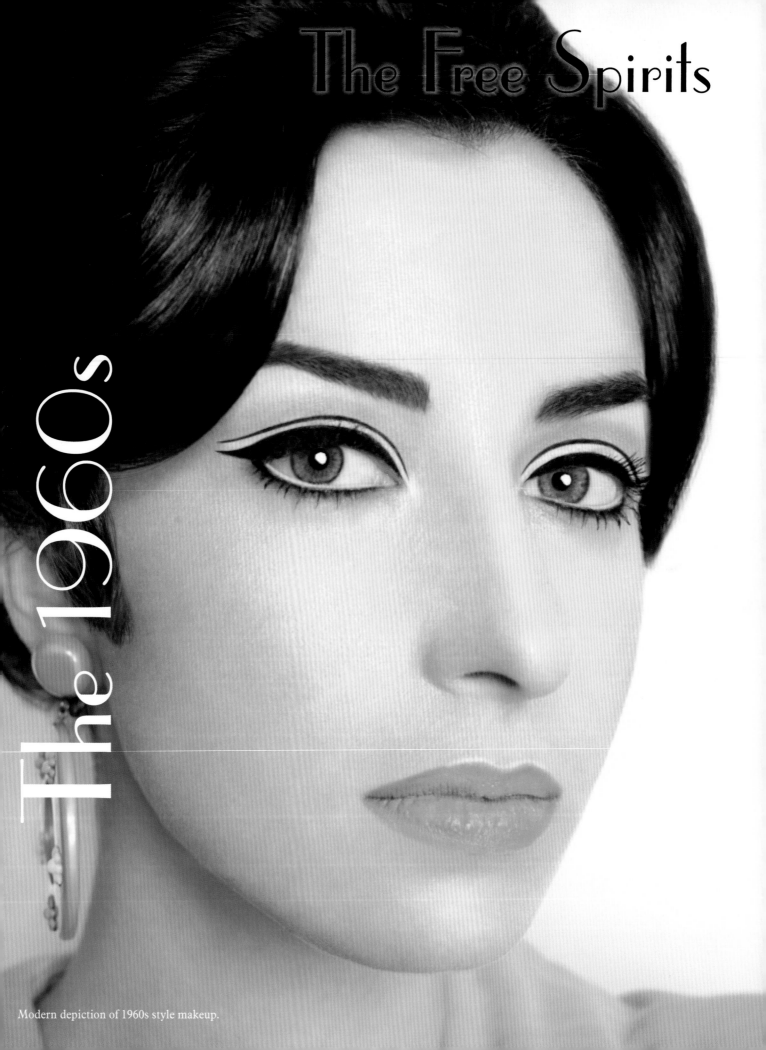

The 1960s

Modern depiction of 1960s style makeup.

The fashion and style of the 1950s was prosperous, prim, and modest, informed by Parisian chic. When America's youngest President, John Fitzgerald Kennedy, took office in 1961, this upbeat trend seemed destined to continue forever. President Kennedy's tragic assassination in 1963 exposed a smoldering dark side to the American dream. This national restlessness was already present in cinema's leading men of the time, like the troubled James Dean (*Rebel Without a Cause*) and the brooding Marlon Brando (*A Streetcar Named Desire*, *The Wild One*, and *On the Waterfront*). In music, Elvis Presley was undeniably sexy, but heavy and moody. With the Beatles' 1964 American debut on The Ed Sullivan Show, the so-called British Invasion that launched a decades-long youth quake was underway.

Paris may have been the couture capital for the old guard, but swinging London became the irreverent epicenter of pop culture in the 1960s. Vidal Sassoon, a London hairdresser, triggered waves of consumer trends with his revolutionary haircuts. Prior to Sassoon, the women he called his "grannies" had kept to a pre-war schedule of a salon wash and roller-set every two weeks or so, the finished result being a rigid, sprayed updo. Feeling the zeitgeist of generational change, Sassoon instead challenged women to pull out the hairpins, rinse out the lacquer and allow their hair to comply with gravity, cutting the hair to fall naturally at lengths from the chin to shoulder. This radical approach made the salon visit only an occasional necessity, for cut and color; women could shampoo and style at home. The ingenious Sassoon and his myriad imitators quickly formulated and marketed retail shampoos, conditioners, and styling products for what he termed "wash and wear hair," thus creating a lucrative new industry.

Liberation from ritual defined the 1960s. London-based designer and makeup innovator Mary Quant claimed that she created the first miniskirt for herself, so she could run for the bus. With perfect synergy, pantyhose (in natural colors as well as wild patterns) hit the market, replacing bulky garters. As in the 1920s, a slim, boyish body came to symbolize the free-wheeling times, and no one epitomized this more than Twiggy, born Lesley Hornby, the first international supermodel so-named for her natural slenderness. Just as Sassoon's snipped, geometric haircuts became a generational shorthand, Twiggy's eye-makeup became the standard, including drawing tiny lines with liquid liner between the lower lashes to make the eyes seem wider and more waif-like. Twiggy herself was still a dewy-skinned 17-year-old when she was proclaimed "The Face of 1966."

Live music and late-night clubs became the throbbing, groovy heart of London in the 1960s, and fashion and style worldwide were imprinted with Cockney accents, Carnaby Street flash, and the tempo of the Mersey Beat. Twiggy's slightly androgynous look was in key with the times: English rock royalty, beginning with The Rolling Stones' Mick Jagger and Keith Richards and followed by the even more outlandish David Bowie and many others, wore makeup onstage and off. The message was androgynous, erotic, exotic, and confrontational. Bowie in particular took inspiration from the ongoing "space race," styling his intergalactic Ziggy Stardust appearance after a "Star Man."

Based on the explosive success of the Beatles, marketers of every stripe flooded American consciousness with products intended for teenage girls. The youth market became the most powerful phenomenon in the history of manufacturing, pushed to new heights by technology: jet travel, television, expanded reach of radio broadcasting. The music industry, far more so than motion pictures, became the primary marketing medium used to reach the teen market. As a flowering of the British Invasion, exotic-seeming products and packaging, which suggested the Spice Route and Silk Road, found an instant audience among young Americans. One immediate expression of this was the cat's eye or heavily-lined, Egyptian-style eyeliner as worn not only by Keith Richards, but also by Cher and Barbra Streisand, whose obvious ethnicity defied the WASPy, All-American beauty standard of the 1950s.

Back in the USA, the Beach Boys sang angelic harmonies about surfer girls, summer loves, hot rods, and perfect tans. Surf culture spawned the popularity of home self-blonding, with hair-bleaching and highlighting kits like "Sun In" and "Frost & Tip." In spite of grassroots resistance to America's involvement in the Vietnam War, and simmering racial violence, which peaked with the assassination of the activist Reverend Dr. Martin Luther King Jr. in 1968, the decade ended on a note of innocence and hope: Woodstock.

Did the Beatles wear wigs, as rumor had it? No, they did not. But false hair was all the rage, as girls wore wigs to reinvent their personalities and looks. Women achieved an ethereal look with short hair and a sexy mod look with long locks and full bangs. At the beginning of the decade, the ideal face was permanently young, with wide eyes, pale skin, and pale frosted lips. The end of the decade turned to exotic colors and body painting.

Large darkened eyes were much more pronounced than in the '50s. Lipstick came in shades like Beach Peach, Swinging Pink, and Little Red. Neutral shades were more popular than bright reds. Rouge was now called blusher, and it was used heavily in earthy brown shades placed under the cheekbones to create shadows to alter the face's shape. False lashes were immensely popular, starting with a version applied in single lashes and moving to the row styles used today. They were manufactured with sable, mink, or human hair, and eventually produced in outrageous colors like foils and tweeds.

Leg makeup was popular again due to the use of the mini skirt. A complete range of products designed for the legs included tinted powder and rouge for the knees. Some of the early body bronzers turned the skin orange and created an uneven blotchy finish when applied on dry skin areas.

Shadow colors were offered in sets. Cream color shadows came in disposable plastic tubes. Metallics were added to many products for the eyes, lips, and face.

With the Catholic Church's acceptance of plastic surgery for extreme cases of disfigurement or the necessity of certain lines of work, the subject of plastic surgery was discussed openly amongst women.

In spite of the prominence of diversity, Elizabeth Arden popularized an arctic look for blondes, and released a Swedish collection of skincare aimed at the light skinned customers.

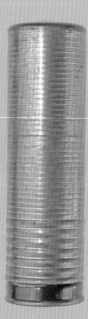

Elizabeth Arden Regal
Red lipstick, c. 1962.

Decade Highlights

- Helena Rubinstein invents waterproof mascara.
- The pill is introduced in 1960.
- Mary Quant designs the most important fashion item of the decade, the mini skirt. She personifies the London look of the 1960s and revolutionizes the face of British fashion. Her first USA tour accompanied by leggy models, stops traffic on Broadway.
- The beehive hairstyle is popular in the beginning of the decade. It is later replaced by the geometric styles of Vidal Sassoon.
- Helen Gurley Brown, future editor of *Cosmopolitan* magazine, publishers her bombshell book *Sex and the Single Girl*.
- Germaine Monteil liquid blusher and Hazel Bishop Fresh'n'Bright blusher are produced in 1963, remaining popular until the 1980s.
- Russian Valentina Tereshkova is the first woman sent into orbit in 1963.
- The Civil Rights Movement intensifies with Martin Luther King Jr.'s march on Washington in 1963.
- Yves Saint-Laurent launches Rive Gauche fragrance in 1968.
- The Beatles visit Maharishi in 1968, which makes trips to India and a communion with nature fashionable.
- Neil Armstrong takes the first walk on the moon in 1969.
- Custom beauty counters are introduced where women can play with makeup and experiment with new looks.
- Mary Quant introduces Jeeper Peepers mascara in several colors and a half and half lipstick called Skitso.
- Revlon develops the first hypo-allergenic department store line of products called Etherea.
- "Everyone will be famous for fifteen minutes." Andy Warhol.

The Face

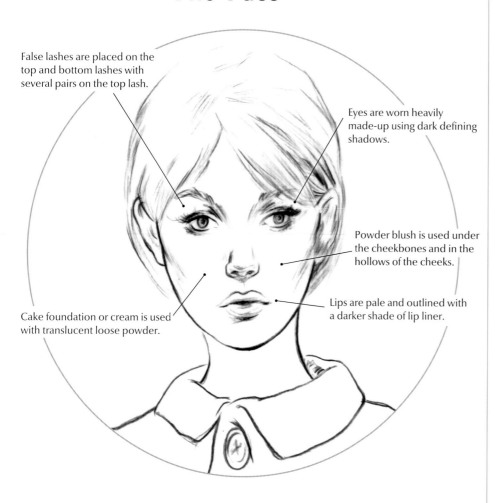

False lashes are placed on the top and bottom lashes with several pairs on the top lash.

Eyes are worn heavily made-up using dark defining shadows.

Powder blush is used under the cheekbones and in the hollows of the cheeks.

Cake foundation or cream is used with translucent loose powder.

Lips are pale and outlined with a darker shade of lip liner.

Penelope Tree, English fashion model, inspired the swinging '60s movement, photo c. 1960s.

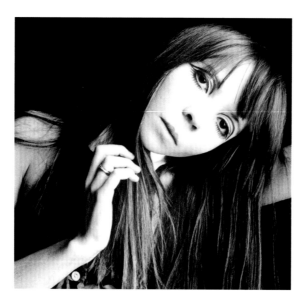

COLOR PALETTE of the 1960s

CAKE

Flesh

CREAM

Tan

POWDER

Translucent

BLUSHER

Soft Rose

Warm Brown

SHADOW

White/Pink

Aqua

Green

Blue

Brown

LINER

Brown/Black

LIQUID LINER

Black

LIPSTICK

Peach

Frost

Pink

The 1960s Face
Emphasis on the Eyes

Eyebrows are left more natural and lightly feathered.

Eyes are emphasized with heavy shadows and thick liners. False lashes in thicker styles are popular for the top and bottom of the eye. Roll-on mascara in black or brown is introduced at this time, and a heavy application on the top and bottom lashes is in fashion. The eyelid wears heavy liner on top and bottom, and a defined shadow is applied in the socket. Later, Twiggy popularizes drawing lashes under the eyes.

Lips are kept pale with shades of peach and outlined with a darker pencil. The lips are slightly overdrawn and finished with gloss in a pearly shade. In frosty sheer pastels, Yardley Pot 'o Gloss, the first lip gloss of its kind versus a hard stick, was marketed aggressively on television during the broadcast of *The Monkees*, popular with tween and pre-teen girls.

A natural foundation that matches the color of the skin is used. Darker foundations are created to match sun tanned skin.

The term rouge loses favor, and is re-named blusher. A tan brown shade under the cheekbones is worn to contour the face.

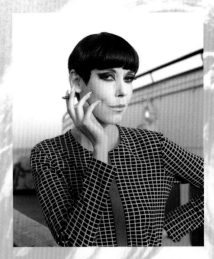

Peggy Moffitt, top American fashion model, October 1965.

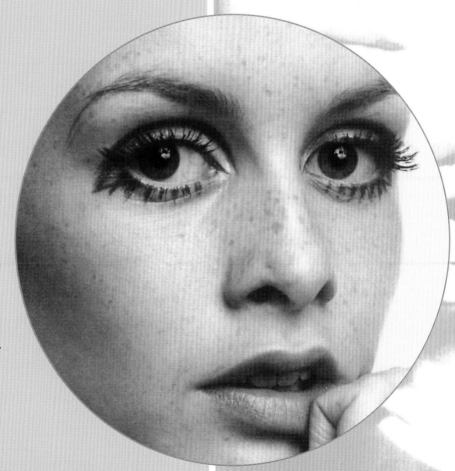

Twiggy, English model and actress, photo c. mid-1960s.

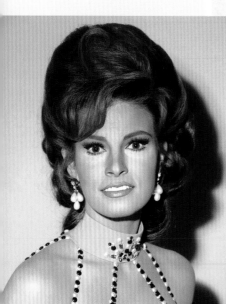

Raquel Welch, U.S. film actress, c. 1965.

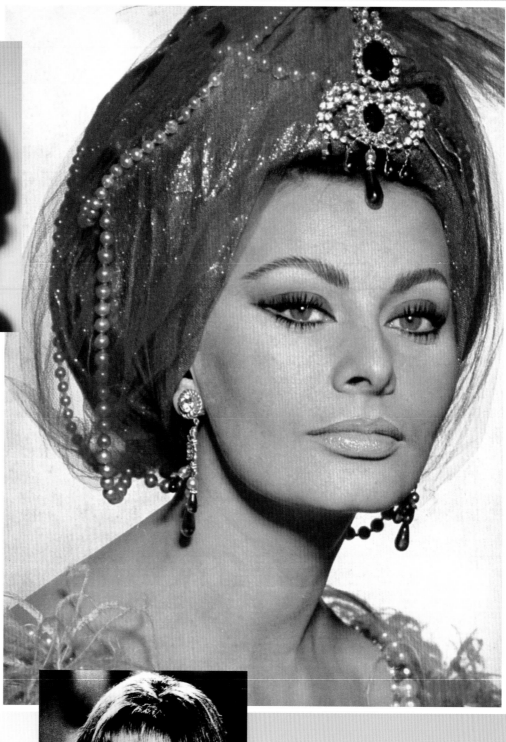

Sophia Loren, Italian screen goddess, photo 1965.

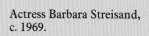

Actress Barbara Streisand, c. 1969.

144

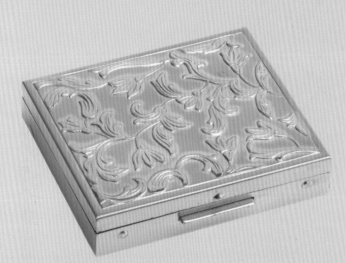

Borden Co. Marcelle powder in Shade #1 and lipstick in Pearle Pink, 1960.

Flower embossed metal compact, refillable for loose powder, c. late 1960s.

Angel Face brand face powder advertisement, model Jean Shrimpton, 1963.

THE LOOK IS FRESH...NATURAL...UTTERLY HEAVENLY

...SO PUT ON YOUR *Angel Face*

... and you'll look radiant as an angel. Angel Face is the complete make-up ... powder and foundation in-one ... that covers every tiny freckle and flaw. Angel Face Make-up holds light to give your face a look that's sheer heaven. In 8 heavenly shades. From 69¢ to $1.25 plus tax.

Angel Face

COMPACT MAKE-UP

Her lipstick is Pink Sugar by Angel Face.

Foundation

A Max Factor cake foundation or cream is a popular choice to use. Translucent loose powder is adopted by consumers when models and film stars make it popular during fashion shoots.

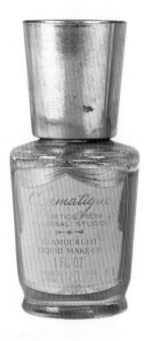

Cinematique brand liquid makeup, 1966.

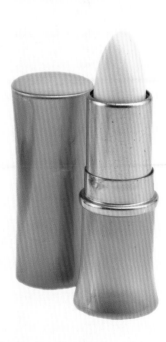

Borden Co. Marcelle lipstick in Pearle Pink, 1960.

Blush

Powder blush is applied under the cheekbones and in the hollows of the cheeks. Warm brown is heavily applied. A narrow triangle of blush under the cheekbones extends to the side of the face.

Eyes

Eyes are worn heavily made-up with dark, defined shadows. A base of white shadow is applied in a powder or cream stick from the lashes to the brow. Aqua, green, or blue shadow is then applied to the lid.

The crease of the eye is darkened with a defined half crescent shape placed over the eye socket. Fashion forward women wear black liner, while more elegant women wear brown-black. Liner is drawn as an elongated triangle from the corner of the eye. It extends out past the end of the eye. A bottom liner is added that follows the same shape and does not meet with the top liner, but is perpendicular to it.

False lashes are placed on the top and bottom lashes, sometimes using several pairs on the top lash. They are coated with black or brown-black mascara. Later on in the decade, British model Twiggy influences the look of lower lashes that are drawn on the skin with black pencil.

Eyebrows are left natural and feathered with a light brown powder shadow.

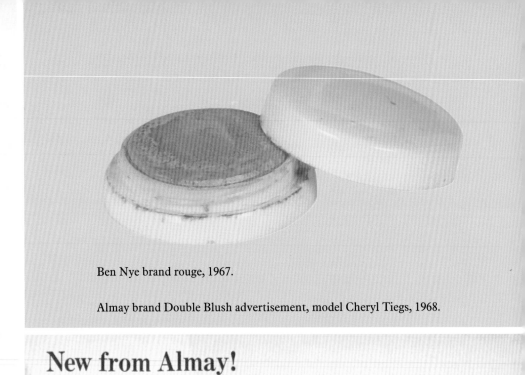

Ben Nye brand rouge, 1967.

Almay brand Double Blush advertisement, model Cheryl Tiegs, 1968.

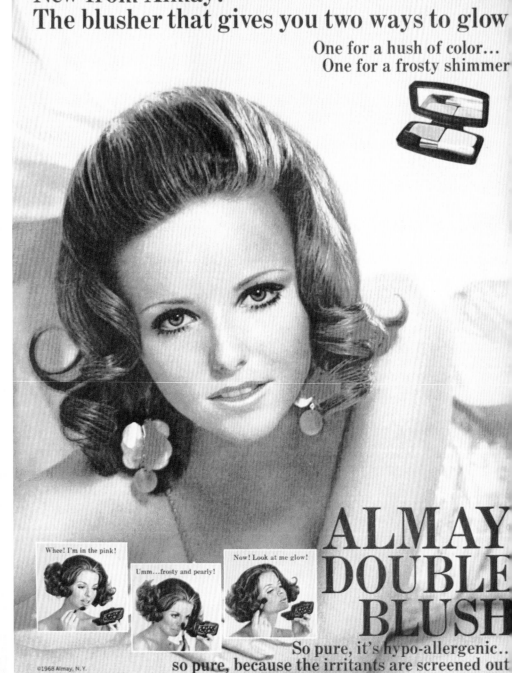

New from Almay!
The blusher that gives you two ways to glow

One for a hush of color...
One for a frosty shimmer

Whee! I'm in the pink!

Umm...frosty and pearly!

Now! Look at me glow!

ALMAY
DOUBLE
BLUSH

So pure, it's hypo-allergenic...
so pure, because the irritants are screened out

©1968 Almay, N.Y.

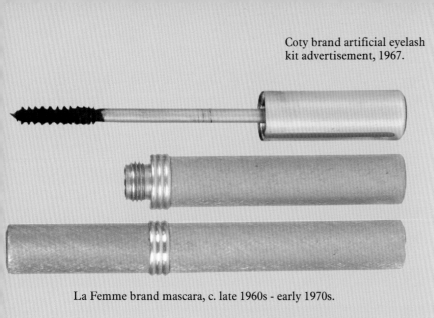

Coty brand artificial eyelash kit advertisement, 1967.

La Femme brand mascara, c. late 1960s - early 1970s.

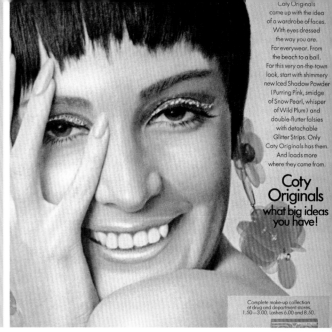

Coty Originals came up with the idea of a wardrobe of faces. With eyes dressed the way you are. For everywear. From the beach to a ball. For this very on-the-town look, start with shimmery new Iced Shadow Powder (Purring Pink, smidge of Snow Pearl, whisper of Wild Plum) and double-flutter falsies with detachable Glitter Strips. Only Coty Originals has them. And loads more where they came from.

Coty Originals what big ideas you have!

Complete make-up collection at drug and department stores. 1.50—3.00. Lashes 6.00 and 8.50.

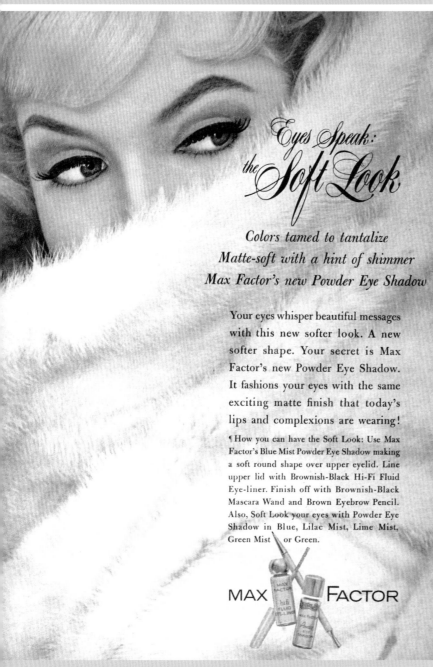

Eyes Speak: the *Soft Look*

Colors tamed to tantalize
Matte-soft with a hint of shimmer
Max Factor's new Powder Eye Shadow

Your eyes whisper beautiful messages with this new softer look. A new softer shape. Your secret is Max Factor's new Powder Eye Shadow. It fashions your eyes with the same exciting matte finish that today's lips and complexions are wearing!

¶ How you can have the Soft Look: Use Max Factor's Blue Mist Powder Eye Shadow making a soft round shape over upper eyelid. Line upper lid with Brownish-Black Hi-Fi Fluid Eye-liner. Finish off with Brownish-Black Mascara Wand and Brown Eyebrow Pencil. Also, Soft Look your eyes with Powder Eye Shadow in Blue, Lilac Mist, Lime Mist, Green Mist or Green.

MAX FACTOR

Max Factor brand Soft Look eye shadow advertisement, 1961.

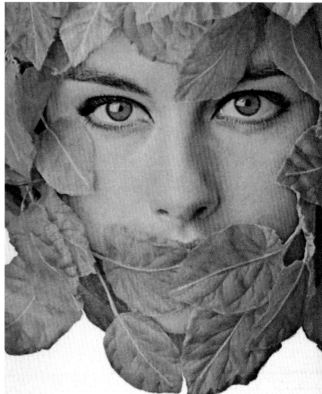

If Eve had worn <u>Aziza</u>, she wouldn't have needed an apple

The ever-so-innocent, irresistible look of Eve. Shimmery, shadow-y lids and lashes, color-kissed with three lovely eye-ssentials from Aziza—Creme Stick Eye Shadow, Waterproof Brush-On Mascara, Liquid Lid Liner. Eve wears greens. What shades for you? Misty blues, delicate purples, velvety browns? For new loveliness, look for Aziza on fine cosmetic counters everywhere.

from PRINCE MATCHABELLI

Aziza brand eye cosmetics advertisement, 1966.

EYES by *Aziza*

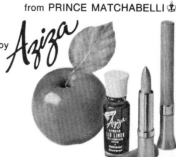

Lips

Lips are generally light in color. To define the shape of the lips, they are outlined with a darker shade of lip liner. The top lip is slightly overdrawn at the corners and filled in with a pale pink or peach lipstick. Gloss is used in pale colors or clear.

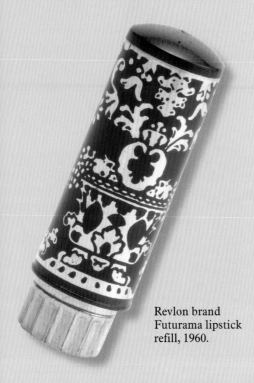

Revlon brand Futurama lipstick refill, 1960.

Coty brand Cremestick lipstick advertisement, 1966.

Max Factor brand California Colors Galore lipsticks with matching nail polishes advertisement, 1963.

Nails

Nails are kept light and painted with white opaque nail enamels.

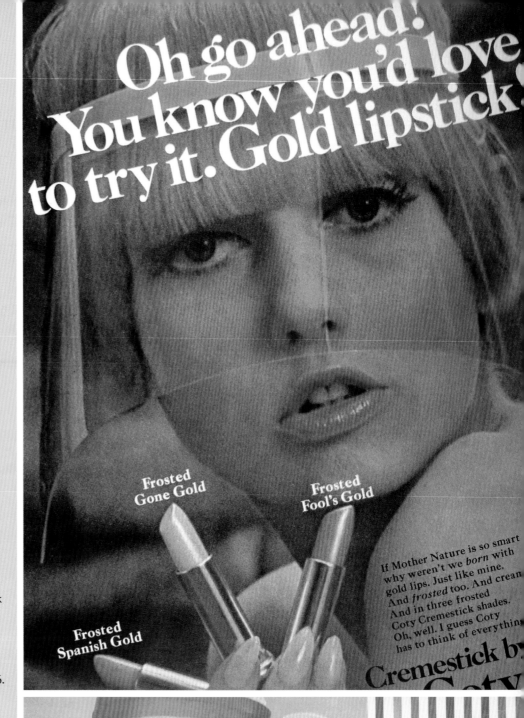

Oh go ahead! You know you'd love to try it. Gold lipstick

Frosted Gone Gold

Frosted Fool's Gold

Frosted Spanish Gold

If Mother Nature is so smart why weren't we *born* with gold lips. Just like mine. And *frosted* too. And cream. And in three frosted Coty Cremestick shades. Oh, well. I guess Coty has to think of everythin

Cremestick by Coty

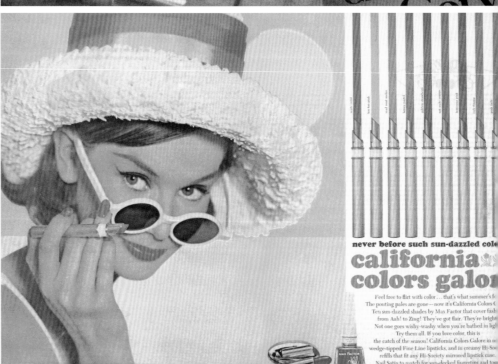

never before such sun-dazzled colo

california colors galor

Feel free to flirt with color... that's what summer's fo
The pouting pales are gone—now it's California Colors C
Ten sun-dazzled shades by Max Factor that cover fash
from Aah! to Zing! They've got flair. They're brigh
Not one goes wishy-washy when you're bathed in ligh
Try them all. If you love color, this is
the catch of the season! California Colors Galore is i
wedge-tipped Fine Line lipsticks, and its creamy Hi-So
refills that fit any Hi-Society mirrored lipstick ca
Nail Satin to match for sun-decked fingertips and t

Marlo Thomas, star of the TV show *That Girl*. Thomas was an early feminist, and her perky character Anne-Marie, an independent young woman on her own in New York City, was considered groundbreaking, c. 1967.

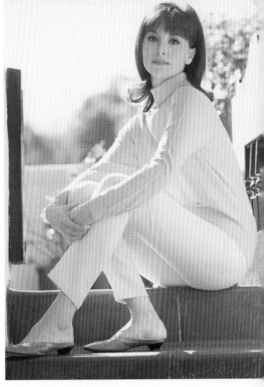

Max Factor pop-up lipstick case. Metal with embossed flowers, c. 1960s.

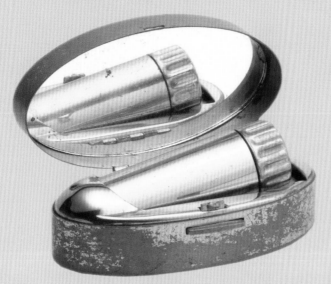

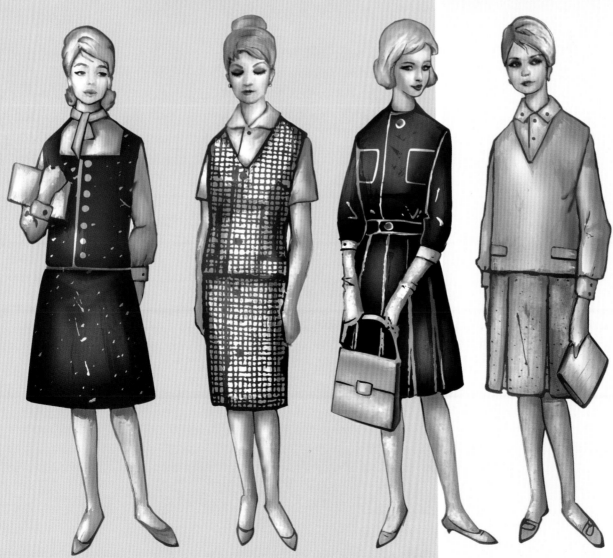

Fashion looks of the 1960s.

Historical TIMELINE

A.D. 1977 to A.D. 2002

1983
Collagen and silicone are first used for cosmetic purposes to create new skin for burn victims.

1985
The cosmetics industry represents 2 billion in annual sales in the United States.

1984
M•A•C brand cosmetics is founded.

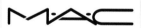

1977
Fiberglass nails become an alternative to acrylics.

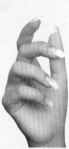

1988
The L'Oréal company acquires Helena Rubinstein, one of the pioneering cosmetics brands in the United States.

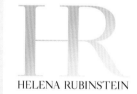

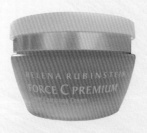

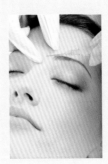

1995
Chemists stabilize
vitamin C.
Helena Rubinstein
introduces Force C
facial cream.

1998
Sephora opens in
New York, bringing
prestige brands to the
self-service beauty
counter.

FDA approves
Botox for
cosmetics use on
frown lines and
it becomes the
hottest trend for
temporary wrinkle
reduction.

1996
L'Oréal USA, Inc.
acquires Maybelline.

2002
Self tanning cubicles
become more available and
customers are sprayed with
a bronzer that gives off a
more even tan in less than 5
minutes.

1991
Colored
acrylics for nails
are introduced
and allow
customers to
go without nail
polish.

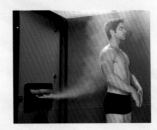

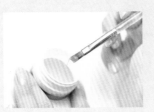

Disco, Punk & Endless Summer

The 1970s

Modern depiction of 1970s style makeup.

The 1970s dawned with the rising of a dark star. Just a few months after Woodstock, a Rolling Stones show in Altamont, California, made world headlines not for its music but for a murder and the accidental deaths of other concertgoers. While flower children still carried on the optimism of the Age of Aquarius, a harder, metallic attitude settled over America. At its heart was deep political cynicism, which peaked during the Watergate hearings, a scandal which drove maligned President Richard M. Nixon out of office in disgrace in 1974.

Still, the party raged on. The shimmery center of world nightlife moved to Manhattan's Studio 54, which drew the world's most beautiful people and the most ravaged celebrity attention seekers. The music was coldly synthetic, pumping out a relentless disco beat. Fashions were clingy, silky, silvery, and slippery. The dance floor was dominated by the slick and slinky moves of the hustle, the New York hustle, and the Latin hustle, along with other complex, highly choreographed standards—so different from the freestyle wiggling of Woodstock. The decade's soundtrack was the facile funk of The Bee Gees, and the porn-star gasps and sighs of diva Donna Summers, sounds which dominated glossy, high-end gyms like Equinox, which became the era's hottest nightspots for mingling and being seen as well as pumping iron.

The propriety of the 1950s was mocked as false. Americans across all generations were dispirited, and felt betrayed by the government in which their parents had believed so righteously. When the USA evacuated the last remaining American troops from Vietnam in 1973, the lingering aftermath of scars began. To counteract the climate of growing hopelessness, activism of all kinds flowered. Feminism, as led by Gloria Steinem, Betty Freidan, and Germaine Greer, operated on the belief that "A woman without a man is like a fish without a bicycle."

The vision and knowledge of Steinem contributed to less politically militant pop culture interpretations of feminism, such as the television show *That Girl*, starring Marlo Thomas, the availability of the Pill, and the publication of *Cosmopolitan* editor, Helen Gurley Brown's, astonishing book *Sex and the Single Girl* a decade earlier.

All of this gave fire not only to the feminist movement, but to the beauty industry and to the manufacturers of cosmetics as well. The word was out: looking pretty and sexy did not mean that you were not a liberated woman. In the 1970s, women did indeed push back against long-standing norms revered by their mothers' generation. For instance, "hot pants"—the name alone connoted a high libido back in the 1920s—or super short-shorts that became acceptable public attire in the 1970s. Nudity in varying degrees, including nudity in movies, grew more palatable. Some women protested pre-liberation standards of beauty by refusing to shave their underarms or legs, though most continued the traditional practice of depilation.

An icon of the 1970s was the long, leggy model-actress Shelly Hack, striding through the television and print ads for Revlon's "Charlie," a best-selling fragrance. She was the newest incarnation of Katharine Hepburn's distinctly un-frilly roles from three decades earlier, hands in her trouser pockets, confident, and irresistible. This attitude was a radical departure from the way that women were traditionally portrayed in fragrance ads just a generation earlier, usually as swooning, virginal doves or devilish temptresses. The independent woman was conscious of her body and strove to maintain it well. There were many diets and exercise programs to try, as well as a new crop of diet products. Like the disco, the din at gyms and health clubs opening all across the country was deafening. Disco hits pounded the walls as patrons felt the burn and the exercise craze made the warm-up suit popular. The suits and their matching headbands came in all colors. They were made primarily of polyester, the new wrinkle-free fabric of the decade. Other trends such as jersey wrap dresses, pantsuits, and tight designer jeans were tailor made to flatter a svelte figure.

The era of the strong woman fit very well with fashion models who weren't just known for their pretty faces. They spoke on current issues such as conservation and health issues, and helped with philanthropic causes. Marisa Berenson, Lauren Hutton, Margaux Hemingway, Cheryl Tiegs, and Christie Brinkley had the healthy and athletic look companies were willing to pay for. In 1972, Hutton earned a staggering $175,000 per year to promote the Ultima II cosmetics line.

Popularized by actress and '70s TV star Farrah Fawcett, her blonde, rough cut, flicked, and feathered hairstyle became the iconic hairdo of the decade. Her posters sold millions of copies and inspired all kinds of hair and cosmetics products. Constant use of blow drying, tongs, or heated rollers were required to make the hair flick for a natural, carefree look. Other styles included Afro perms that only required washing and forking with a special lifting and separating comb. Another popular hairstyle created by Trevor Sorbie in 1974 was immortalized by figure skater Dorothy Hamill after her gold medal win at the 1976 Olympics. Her short bobbed hairstyle, dubbed the Hamill Wedge, became a look that is forever tied to the 1970s.

Relaxation and natural remedies were found to improve the skin. Botanical formulas were introduced in France and made their way to the U.S. in the form of aromatherapy. Wheat germ and hops serums, seaweed baths and lily based makeup were introduced. Other products made from coconut oil and flower extracts claimed to provide the skin with a self-protection system, and caviar eggs had stimulating effects on the skin.

With Chanel and Yves Saint-Laurent leading the way, the major couture houses of Europe entered the cosmetics field. They brought creamier, smoother textures and bolder colors to their lipsticks. Some lipsticks even featured a sun protection filter.

Punk and metal bands were the nihilistic dark side of the Age of Aquarius. Punk bands like Sex Pistols, Clash, and Black Flag, , as well as metal bands like Megadeath, Iron Maiden, and Def Leppard inspired young people to shed their home-grown hippie regalia for buzzed hair, black leather clothes, and skin ritually pierced and stabbed by multiple, anarchy-inciting safety pins.

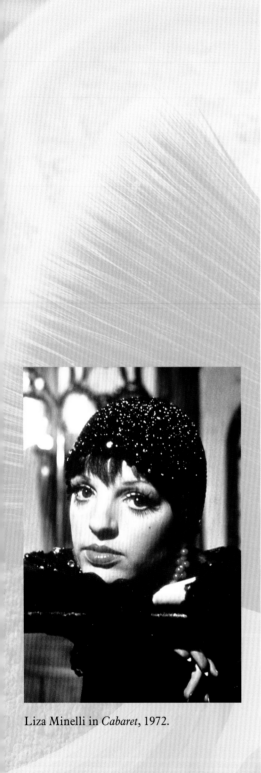

Liza Minelli in *Cabaret*, 1972.

Decade Highlights

- Hair products such as Elnett hair spray and Petrole Hahn Lotion flood the market.
- Cosmetic surgery, notably the nose job and the face lift, become available to the masses.
- Botanical medicine and aromatherapy coming from France become popular, leading to the popularity of seaweed baths, wheat germ, and lily based makeup.
- New York makeup artist Trish McEvoy identifies a void in the huge cosmetics industry of quality application tools. She creates professional quality makeup brushes and mass markets them to the consumer.
- Patrick Alés creates Phytoplage, a line of hair products for the sun.
- Bill Gates and Paul Allen start Microsoft in 1975.
- Apple Computer Inc. is founded in 1976.
- Clarins develops bust-care products.
- In 1977, *Star Wars* captures the imagination of millions and revolutionizes special effects for motion pictures.
- YSL introduces a makeup line in 1978.
- Estée Lauder introduces Re-Nutriv cream, a light formula with sun block.
- "There are no ugly women, there are only women who do not know themselves." Marcella Borghese

The Face

Shimmer shadows are used on the eye lids with mascara on the top and bottom lashes.

Eyebrows are kept natural, brushed, and tamed with clear mascara.

Light liquid formulas and opalescent or pearlized powders are used for a healthy glow.

Bronzer powders are applied liberally all over the face; berry shades on the apples of the cheek are meant to look natural.

Shiny clear glosses or pink and nude pearl lipsticks coat the lips.

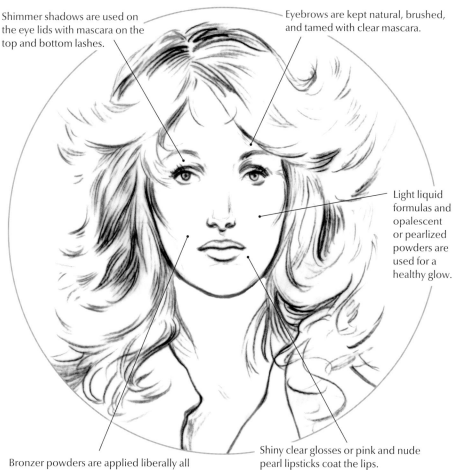

COLOR PALETTE of the 1970s

LIGHT LIQUID

Flesh

LIQUID OR CREAM

Tan

POWDER

Opalescent/ Iridescent

BLUSH

Light Pink

SHADOW

Light Blue

Dark Brown

Lightest Blue

Light Purple Frost

Light Green

LINER

Kohl

LIPSTICK OR LIPGLOSS

Peachy Pink

Pink Frost

Light Peach Frost

Nude Frost

Earth Coral

Fuchsia Gloss

Farrah Fawcett, television star and sex symbol of the '70s, photo 1977.

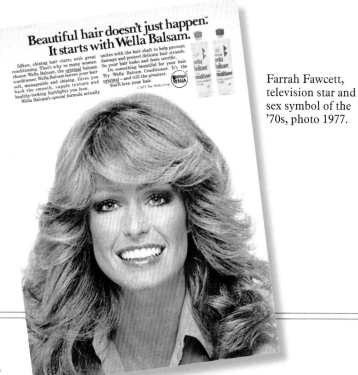

The 1970s Face
Bronzed and Glossed

Women during the '70s worship a tan, athletic, and natural look. They want their looks to be simple and effortless, although it takes more effort than less to achieve this look. Tan brown bronzers are applied liberally to the face to give a sun kissed look.

Shimmers are used to highlight the cheekbones. Natural peaches and pinks are used on the apples of the cheeks. A natural sheer foundation that matches the color of the skin is used. The application is kept light to look natural.

The decade's most characteristic shadow is a fusion of the banana shape over the eyelid crease with the upper lid outlined with shadow. One of the most trend-setting innovations is doing this kind of shading in black and white.

Cream shadows also make their first appearance. The eyelid wears heavy shadows in three coordinating shades, with shimmers becoming very popular.

Rouge begins to be worn in "L" shapes.

The false lashes that appeared in the '60s are also popular in the '70s, but have longer, more natural shapes. These thin, natural styles are popular for the top of the eye and outer corner.

The lips are kept pale with shades of peach and pink for daytime and glossy vibrant colors for evening. Light brown lips, not overly made up, sometimes in the same shade as the foundation, are covered using the very same foundation.

Eyebrows are kept natural and brushed.

Eyes are emphasized with heavy pastel shadows and thick liners in the evening and light to no makeup looks in the daytime.

Mascara in black or brown is applied to look natural for daytime and stronger for evening.

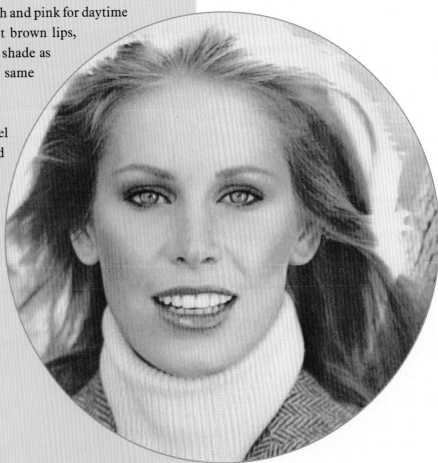

Why do I love Wella Balsam Shampoo? Because it not only conditions your hair. It even helps repair split ends.
—Jaclyn Smith

I used to use an ordinary shampoo. Then I switched to Wella Balsam Shampoo. Because its unique formula not only leaves your hair gloriously clean, it also conditions it. And since I wash my hair every day, that's important. But the thing I love best is that Wella Balsam Shampoo even helps repair split ends. Wella proved that in tests in salons and laboratories.

Between washings, Wella Balsam Shampoo protects your hair from the damage that sun, chlorine, chemicals and pollution can cause. And it gets rid of that fuzzy look. Leaves you with a soft, silken, healthy-looking shine.

Don't settle for an ordinary shampoo. Switch to the shampoo that cleans, conditions and even helps repair split ends. Wella Balsam Shampoo. Regular or new Formula for Oily Hair.

You'll love your hair.

© 1977 The Wella Corp.

Jaclyn Smith, actress and clothing designer, photo 1977.

Cheryl Tiegs, model and actress, photo 1979.

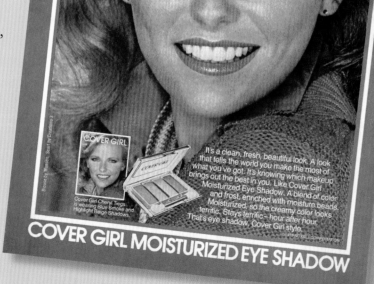

EYE SHADOW, COVER GIRL STYLE

Cover Girl Cheryl Tiegs is wearing Blue Smoke and Highlight Beige Shadows.

It's a clean, fresh, beautiful look. A look that tells the world you make the most of what you've got. It's knowing which makeup brings out the best in you. Like Cover Girl Moisturized Eye Shadow. A blend of color and frost, enriched with moisture beads. Moisturized, so the creamy color looks terrific. Stays terrific—hour after hour. That's eye shadow, Cover Girl style.

COVER GIRL MOISTURIZED EYE SHADOW

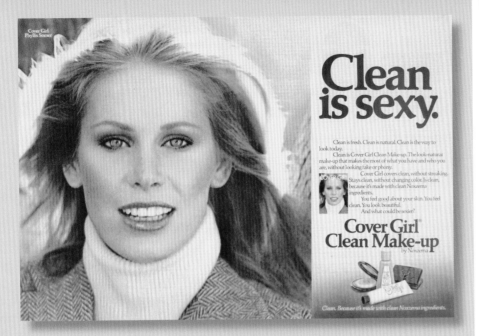

CoverGirl brand Clean Makeup foundation advertisement, 1976.

Foundation

For foundation, a very light application with the use of a liquid formula, is popular for a no makeup look. It is used mainly to even out the skin tone and hide discolorations. Face powders contain opalescent, iridescent, and pearlized pigments to give the face a healthy glow.

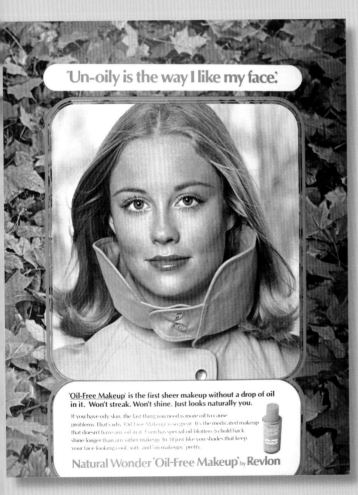

Revlon brand Natural Wonder Oil-Free Makeup advertisement, model Cybill Shepherd, 1971.

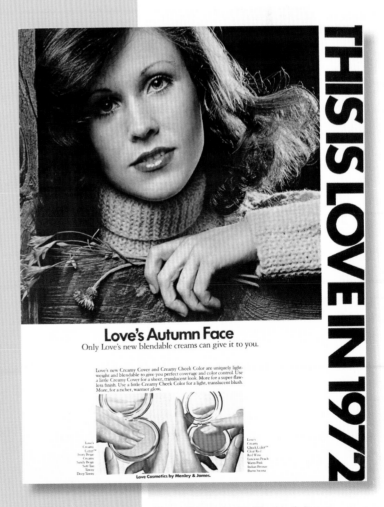

Love Cosmetics by Menley & James brand foundation and cheek color advertisement, 1972.

Blush

Bronzer is applied liberally on the face and well blended. The color is swept with a large brush on the cheekbones, the tip of the nose, chin, jawline, and hairline. The color chosen is two shades darker than the face to maintain a natural look.

Blush is used on the apples of the cheeks. The color is a deeper version of a natural blush, like a vibrant peach or raspberry stain. The color is blended to look like a natural flush. Shimmer highlighter is used on the tops of the cheekbones.

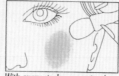
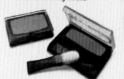
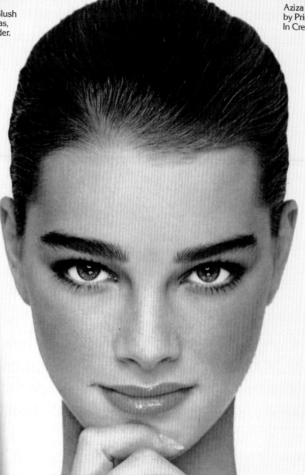

Aziza brand Natural Lustre Blush advertisement, model Brooke Shields, 1979.

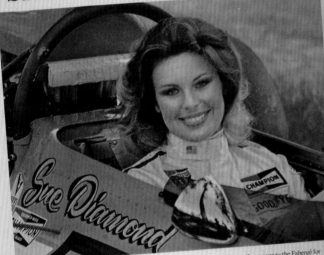
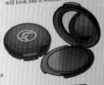
Fabergé brand Compact Cheek Colors blush advertisement, 1975.

Eyes

Eyes feature new shimmer pastel color eye makeup. Black mascara, black eyeliner, and shimmer eye shadows make the eyes very dramatic. During the late '70s, softer looks become more fashionable and replace powders with soft foundations that provide sheer coverage.

The eyes are kept neutral for daytime with mascara used on the top and bottom lashes.

The eyebrows are kept natural, brushed, and tamed with clear mascara. The application is light to look natural. The inner lower lash lines are rimmed with white eye pencil.

For more dramatic and nighttime looks, three highly pigmented shadows in bold colors are applied: one very light and shimmery, the other medium-toned, and the last one is the darkest. They are often different tones of the same shade, such as baby blue, blue-gray, and navy. From lash line to crease, a pearlescent medium shade is used. On the crease and on the outer edges of the upper eyelid, the darkest shadow is used. On the brow bone and inner corner of the eyes, the lightest shade is used. The edges are well blended to fade any hard lines. Pastel shimmer eye shadow is spread on the whole eyelid with an eye shadow brush. The eye is lined underneath with pastel shimmer eye shadow using a small eye shadow brush.

For an evening look, black eyeliner is used on the top eyelid starting at the outside corner of the eye working toward the inside corner of the eye. The line is started high on the outside corner of the eye to achieve a cat-eye look. The bottom of the eye is lined with black eyeliner. Dense false lashes add extra drama to the defined evening makeup.

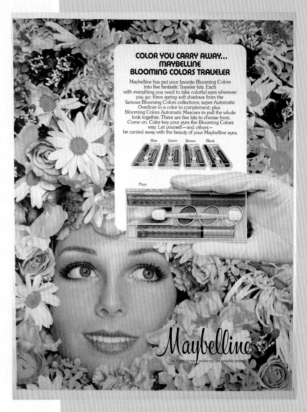

Maybelline brand Blooming Colors Traveler kits advertisement, 1973.

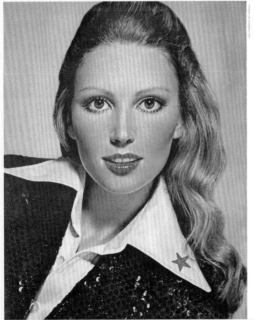

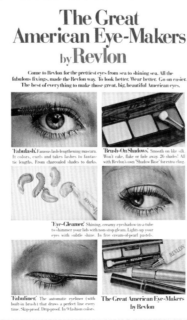

Revlon brand Great American Eye-Makers shadows advertisement, 1971.

161

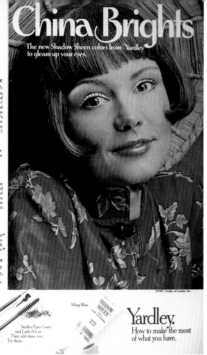

China Brights
The new Shadow Sheen colors from Yardley to gleam up your eyes.

How to make the China Brights Eye.
Revved-up Chinese colors. 5 nifty ones with high-powered luminescent glow. How? Shadow Sheen's a super-frosted eye gel, that's how. For eyes like our girl's, follow these steps. (Substitute other China Brights Colors if you like.)

1. On your eyelids use Mother of Pearl White.

2. Blend China Brights Ming Blue from crease of eye, up toward brow. Stroke Mother of Pearl White under brow to highlight and give your eye an almond-shape effect.

3. Use Panda Black Lash-A-Lot™ mascara. Touch up lashes where mascara often mixes with Panda Black Easy Liner.™

New Shadow Sheen Colors for the China Brights Eye.
- Mother of Pearl White
- Cinnabar Brown
- Lee Chi Amber
- Jade Green

Ming Blue

Yardley Easy Liner and Lash-A-Lot. They add shine, too. Try them.

Yardley.
How to make the most of what you have.

Yardley brand Shadow Sheen and
eye cosmetics advertisement, 1972.

Maybelline brand Eye
Color Styler Pencils
advertisement, 1979.

MEET THE NEW SMOKEYS!

8 smokey shades of Maybelline Eye Color Styler-Pencils

Now write eyes as unique as your signature in 8 new smashing, smokey shades. Line, shadow, contour, style. It's easy with Maybelline Eye Color Styler-Pencils.

Look for all the luscious, blendable colors for eyes and lips! Pick up a bunch and celebrate. *Eye Writing is here!*

GLOWING BRONZE · BROWN BARE · MIDNITE TEAL · BORDEAUX · BURNT CORK · BLAZING GINGER · SMOKEY BEIGE · SMOKEY AMETHYST

Maybelline®
Fine make-up / sensibly priced

© 1979 MAYBELLINE CO.

You're too lib
to live in
anybody's shadow.

Ad lib it
with Yardley Mixis.

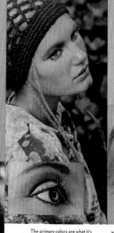

The primary colors are what it's all about.
Tubes of them to play impressionist with. To squeeze. Mix with your fingers. To ad lib your own eye shadow with.
Blue and red to make your own private purple. Add yellow to grow your own green. The works to tie dye. And white to make light of it.
Anything (and everything) to get away from those storebought blues: even a spatula and a paint to pearl with.
All in the Yardley Mixis kit.
All the glorious shadows in the world to ad lib with your fingertips: even if you're all thumbs.

Yardley brand Mixis Finger Mix eye
cosmetics advertisement, 1970.

162

Yardley
You've got to be young to get away with it.

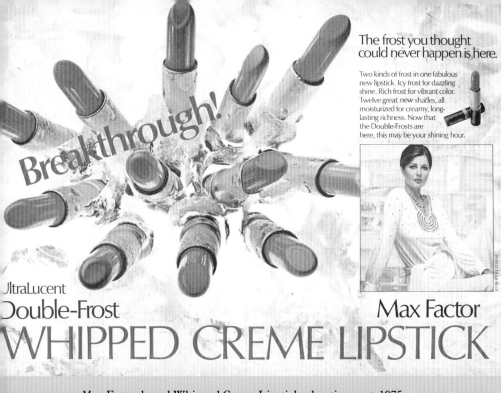

Breakthrough!

UltraLucent
Double-Frost
WHIPPED CREME LIPSTICK

The frost you thought could never happen is here.

Two kinds of frost in one fabulous new lipstick. Icy frost for dazzling shine. Rich frost for vibrant color. Twelve great new shades, all moisturized for creamy, long-lasting richness. Now that the Double-Frosts are here, this may be your shining hour.

Max Factor

Max Factor brand Whipped Creme Lipstick advertisement, 1975.

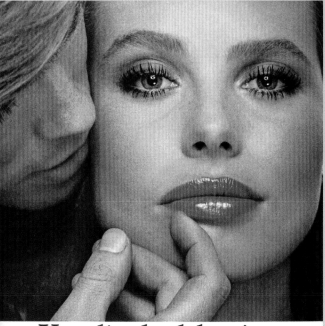

Your lips look luscious, *Babe*

Fabergé introduces the lush, luscious look of creamy Babe Lip Colors. The moist, shiny look of Babe Sheer Lip Glosses. And, lushest of all, Babe clear Liquid Lip Gloss. They all contain sunscreen for added protection. And they're all new from Babe Cosmetics — as fresh, as smart, and as uncomplicated as you are. To help you look fabulous, Babe. *Simply* fabulous.

Babe Cosmetics made fabulous by Faberge Creative Research.

Babe brand cosmetic lip products advertisement, 1977.

Nails

The nails are long and painted with pearls, pastels, and bold color metallics.

Lips

For daytime, a shiny clear gloss or a lip balm the color of the lips is worn. Pink and nude pearl shades are also popular color choices. Lip liners are used to define the shape of the lips.

For a more dramatic look, a glossy lipstick in deep red is used. Deep vibrant jewel tones with a clear gloss on top are used for evening.

Maybelline brand Kissing Potion lip gloss, c. 1970s.

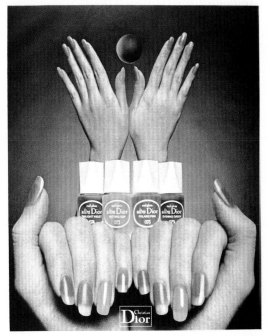

Christian Dior brand Twilight Bright Nail Gloss nail enamel advertisement, 1973.

Shimmering. Shiny. Gleaming nails and lips. Now in soft, clear, twinkling colors of gloss. It's Dior's four new Twilight Bright Nail Gloss and Lip Gloss shades for Spring. Adding new color to your nails and clever new shine to your mouth. There's Polaris Pink. Evening Green. Setting Sun. And Twilight Violet. For a little color or a lot. The more that's added the more the color. Wear one, two, three or more. These are the shades that are made to go with each other, and to go with each of your moods. New Nail Gloss Nail Enamel and Lip Gloss Twilights. All from Christian Dior.

Twilights. Dior.

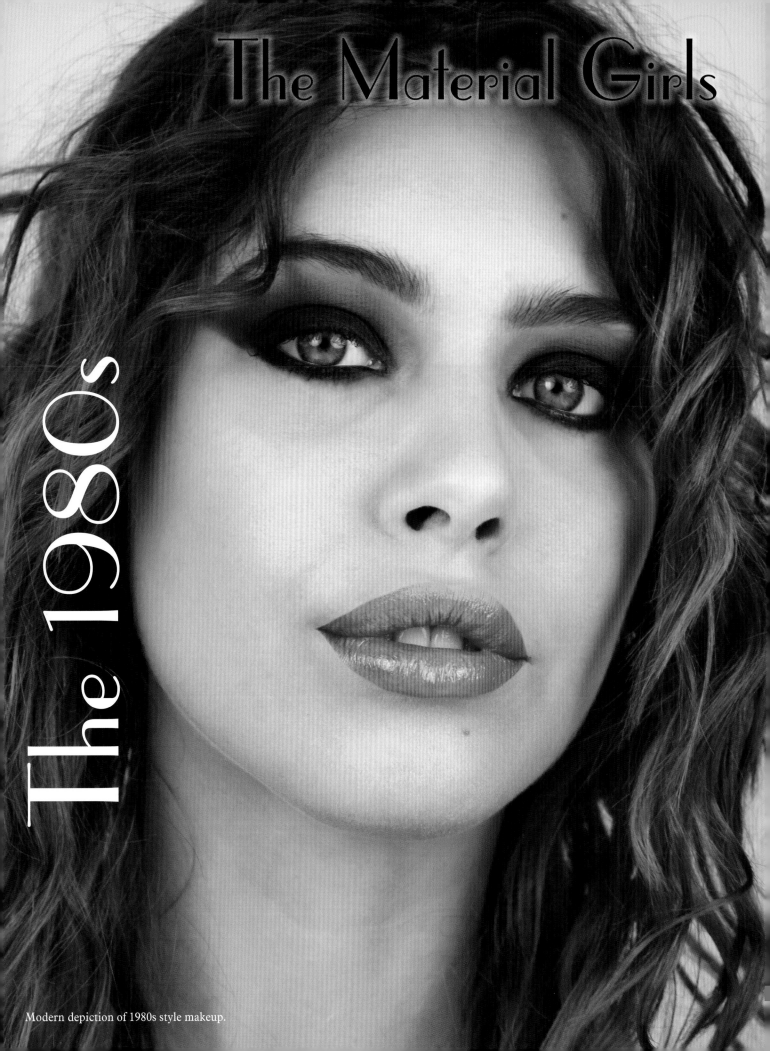

The Material Girls

The 1980s

Modern depiction of 1980s style makeup.

The 1980s was a decade of bold and dramatic trends. Between the last days of the carefree disco movement and a new generation of a rising, female work force, a woman's makeup look tended to be heavy and extreme. She became polished, put together, and powerful. Eighties makeup minimized flaws and accentuated a woman's feminine features with bright blasts of color.

"Nine to Five" became the anthem of the office-bound woman and in the movie *Wall Street*, Gordon Gecko told us "greed is good" and "lunch is for wimps."

In the White House, Ronald Reagan, a former Hollywood screen star, was president. Along with style conscious First Lady Nancy, they brought good looks, glamour, and a sense of abundance to the American people. A well-put together look meant power, and with their perfect appearance, the promise of getting the job done was achievable. His economic policy known as Reaganomics lowered taxes for big business owners and the wealthy class, and assured a trickle down effect for the poor. Credit cards were readily available to consumers, which resulted in an explosion of consumer debt. Going to the mall became a favorite activity and shopping was a national pastime.

Making money was a major concern for many people. MBAs were all the rage in colleges since business jobs offered higher starting salaries. These young urban professionals dubbed "yuppies" were career centered and wanted a high standard of living. Women were also seeking careers, so many couples delayed having children to concentrate on their financial goals. Females assumed the role of a Superwoman. Within the corporate world, they worked their way up to top level positions while also running a household. Crisp business suits in colors from gray to fuchsia, impeccable grooming habits, and layers of luminous makeup defined the look of these female power players. The neutral, natural look was out.

The "preppy look," a retro-inspired trend based on the conservative styles of the 1950s, gave the appearance of wealth in a casual style inspired by the Ivy League and nautical themes from eastern seaboard living. Khakis, shorts, Oxford shirts in plaid prints, and pastel-colored v-neck sweaters were prominent, displaying expensive designer labels such as L.L. Bean, Izod, Ralph Lauren, and Calvin Klein. Oversized clothing, torn shirts, and ragged clothing were trendy options to preppy fashions.

The punk movement of the 1980s continued to develop throughout Europe and New York. These non-conformists craved attention and shocked the public with their combat boots, spike-studded, ripped-up fashions, and violently dyed Mohawk hairdos. Several other styles grew out of the punk movement, including Gothic, which featured a pale complexion and dark lips and eyes, emo (for emotive), and a minimal, synthesizer-laced musical style know as cold wave.

Teenage girls dressed in outrageous looks based on popular movie or music personalities. Madonna and Cyndi Lauper led the way, affecting fashion as well as lifestyle. Carefree and individual, these "Material Girls" set trends with their heavy makeup and layered clothing. Cyndi was known for her extravagant red and orange hairdos that matched her flowing skirts. Madonna became the decade's icon and inspired trends such as lingerie worn as outer wear, crucifixes worn as costume jewelry, heavy shadowed lids, and bleached messy hair with dark roots.

Beauty became a competitive sport, and a woman believed that the body needed to be well toned to get ahead in the world. Being beautiful required work, and women were willing to feel the pain to gain a perfect figure. Physical activity became a necessity as aerobics and jogging were the most popular forms of exercise. The sale of workout VHS tapes exploded, as well as jogging suits and Lycra products. Women squeezed into their tights and frequented gyms, which sprang up all over the United States. Portable music players, like the Sony Walkman, were the perfect accompaniment to the daily jog or workout.

Women also had more access to cosmetic procedures, which saw significant increases by the later part of the decade. Liposuction was a viable and acceptable alternative to acquiring a perfectly sculpted body without diet and exercise.

The push to be healthier brought on an era of low-fat and fat-free food products. Diet products crowded the supermarket shelves. A healthy diet was tied to outer beauty, and nutritional supplements were marketed as a way to keep the skin looking youthful and healthy. Vitamin cocktails were consumed to help delay the aging process.

Hair was big and required the use of many styling products. Teased, permed, and high volume hair styles ruled the worlds of women of all ages from young rebellious teens to career women. On-the-go styles became popular since the corporate world demanded more time from these busy women. Companies responded with many new styling aids and a variety of mousses and sprays to keep hair under control.

Self tanning was in vogue, since it gave people "a healthy glow" and connoted a relaxed, luxurious lifestyle. The Guerlain company led the way with its popular Terracotta line of powder bronzers. This "permanent vacation" look was desired by the many women in stressful corporate jobs.

Supermodels became celebrities in their own right, rivaling some of Hollywood's most famous actors. They had bodies of steel, ample breasts, and luminous skin. Many crossed over and became actresses on the large and small screens. Makeup artists such as Serge Lutens for Shiseido, Terry for Yves Saint-Laurent, and Tyen for Dior became celebrities, since they had the tricks to make any woman beautiful. Many makeup artists became directors at the large fashion houses, designing the color collections for each season.

Larger breasts came back in style, and with this trend came the products to help enhance them. Breast implants became a common procedure. The Clarins brand introduced a firming gel for the bust, and stores carried the first push-up bras called demi-cups. By the end of the 1980s, full curves came back as the most stylish silhouette, replacing the square shoulder pads and narrow waists that were dominant fashion trends.

To aid in the maintenance of youth, creams of all kinds using the latest technological formulas entered the market promising they would prevent wrinkles and combat cellulite. Women demanded more from their makeup, and companies invested more money toward research and development. New anti-aging ingredients were constantly being invented. These active ingredients became available in high-end brands and also drugstore brands, promising more noticeable effects for everyone.

Decade Highlights

- Grace Jones, a surgically enhanced woman, becomes the ultra-female face of the 1980s.
- Ronald Reagan, a former Hollywood screen star, is elected president of the United States in 1980.
- MTV premieres in 1981 and begins the era of the music video and the influence of musicians on fashion and style.
- Compact discs are introduced in 1982.
- Cell phones, although large, heavy, and expensive, become available to the public who could afford them.
- Major beauty brands hire prominent makeup artists as artistic directors.
- Elizabeth Arden launches Lip Fix in 1983, a gel for setting lipstick. It becomes one of the company's best selling products.
- 1984 is "The Year of the Yuppie" as proclaimed by Newsweek magazine.
- Madonna releases the song "Material Girl" in 1985 and establishes a look copied by millions.
- Diane Keaton starred in the Woody Allen classic *Annie Hall* in 1977. Her long limbs, scrubbed skin, plain short hair, and quirky menswear set a generational trend.
- Guerlain introduces Météorites powder in 1987, a product consisting of multicolored spheres that are blended on the skin as they are swirled with a brush.
- Paco Rabanne releases Concentré Actif Restructurant in France in 1987, the first anti-wrinkle products for men.
- Clarins introduces L'Eau Dynamisante, a fragrance marketed for its health benefits. It uses herbs, fruits, and roots to stimulate the senses.
- The Berlin Wall is torn down in November of '89, marking the end of the Cold War.
- "Beauty is an illusion, one any woman can create if she knows how to use makeup to make the magic difference." Betsy Eagles

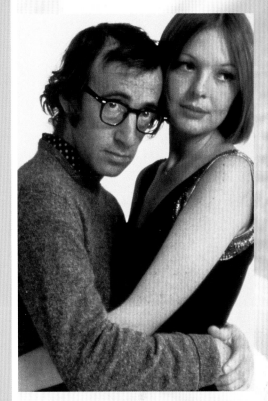

Woody Allen and Diane Keaton in *Annie Hall*, 1977.

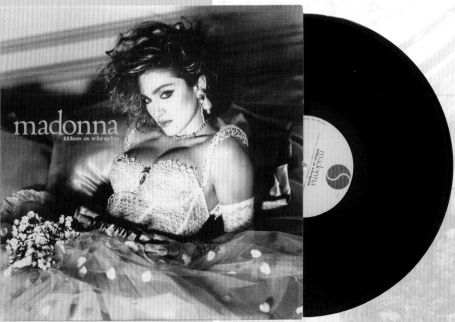

Singer Madonna's second studio album, *Like a Virgin*, 1984.

The Face

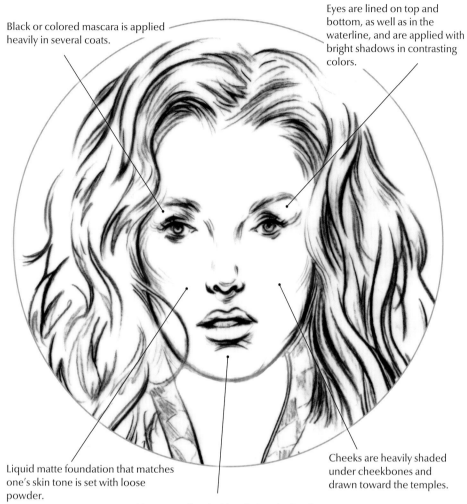

Black or colored mascara is applied heavily in several coats.

Eyes are lined on top and bottom, as well as in the waterline, and are applied with bright shadows in contrasting colors.

Liquid matte foundation that matches one's skin tone is set with loose powder.

Lips are outlined with a darker shade of lip liner and filled in with a bright lipstick.

Cheeks are heavily shaded under cheekbones and drawn toward the temples.

COLOR PALETTE
of the
1980s

LIGHT
LIQUID   POWDER

Flesh   Natural

BLUSH

Brick   Bright Pink
Red

SHADOW

Electric   Shimmer   Frosty
Brown   Lilac

Grass   Pool Blue   Dark   Bright
Green   Frost   Purple   Orange

LINER

Kohl

LIPSTICK

Ultra   Scarlet   Fuchsia
Red

Chocolate   Orange   Mauve
Frost

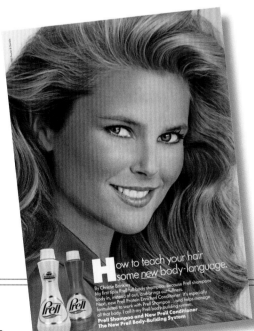

Christie Brinkley, American supermodel, 1985.

The 1980s Face
Big, Bold, and Bright

A rainbow of colors is used on all parts of the face. Makeup companies respond with more color choices and change colors to match the seasons.

Cosmetics companies such as Avon and Mary Kay offer complete makeup kits to take the guess work out of choosing a color scheme.

Lashes are long and painted with green, blue, or black mascara.

The makeup bag of the decade contains a tube of paste-like cover-up, a bottle of heavy foundation, a pressed-powder compact, eye shadows in a rainbow of colors, eyeliner pencils in blue, purple, and teal, blush compacts in pink and brick, mascaras in several shades, and bright lipsticks in shades of red, pink, and orange.

Makeup in the 1980s is a form of war paint for women. They literally "paint" their faces on and wear makeup as a shield. It is a sign of power and control, so more is definitely better.

The two defining makeup elements of the '80s face are bold eyes and a bright stripe of blush that defines the cheek bone.

Eye shadows are bold and bright, and more than one shade is layered to create multicolor effects. The eye shadow color most associated with the '80s is electric blue.

Ultra-red lips accompanied with electric blue shadow and heavily accentuated cheekbones in brick red tones rule the night.

Gloss and everything shiny is popular.

Madonna makes beauty marks popular again. Stick-on beauty marks are available or are simply draw on the skin with brown eyeliner.

Even men use cosmetics. Metal music performers such as Twisted Sister, Mötley Crüe, and Kiss apply cosmetics liberally.

The bright bold patterns and textures in fashion are in stark contrast to the minimal cool, metallic, and modern styles in furniture and interior decor.

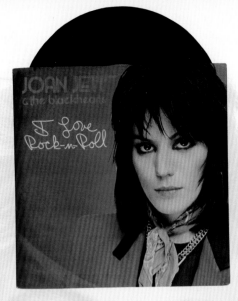

Joan Jett and the Blackhearts, "I Love Rock 'n' Roll" single, 1981.

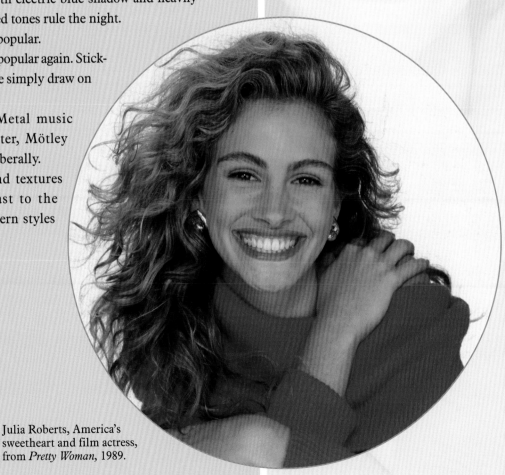

Julia Roberts, America's sweetheart and film actress, from *Pretty Woman*, 1989.

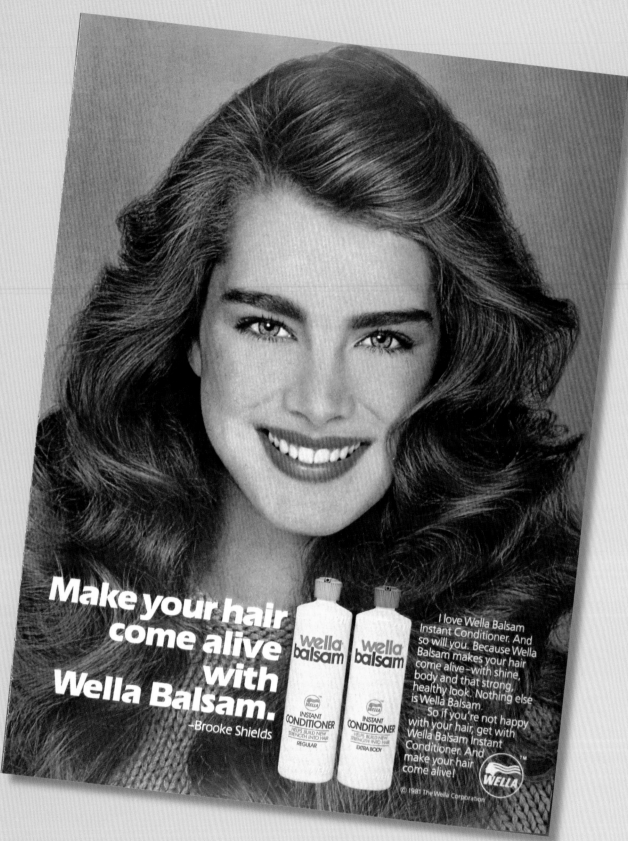

Brooke Shields, model and actress, 1981.

Foundation

The face is cleansed and moisturized. A creamy concealer stick is used around the eye area and to correct any redness. A liquid matte foundation that matches the skin tone is used and blended leaving no line of demarcation. Bronzer is used all over the face for a tanned appearance. Loose powder is used to set the makeup.

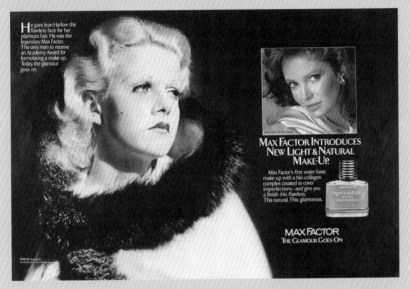

Max Factor brand Light and Natural Makeup foundation advertisement, 1985.

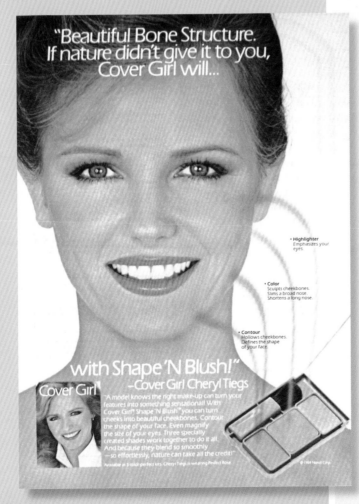

Cover Girl brand Shape 'N Blush advertisement, c. 1984.

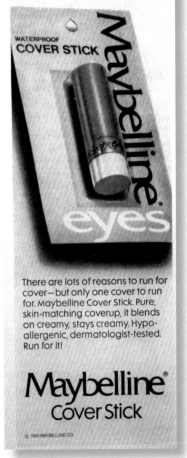

Maybelline brand Cover Stick skin-matching coverup advertisement, 1980.

Blush

Cheeks are heavily shaded under the cheekbone and drawn up toward the temples with bright pink or brick red rouge.

171

Eyes

Eyes are lined on the top and bottom in black, blue, or teal. Liner is also used in the waterline of the eyelids. Fuchsia or bright blue shadow is used on the entire eyelid. Then, a paler or contrasting color such as orange, pink, or white is blended well on the arch of the brow as a highlighter. Black or color mascara is heavily applied in several coats. The brows are left bushy, just lightly groomed and brushed.

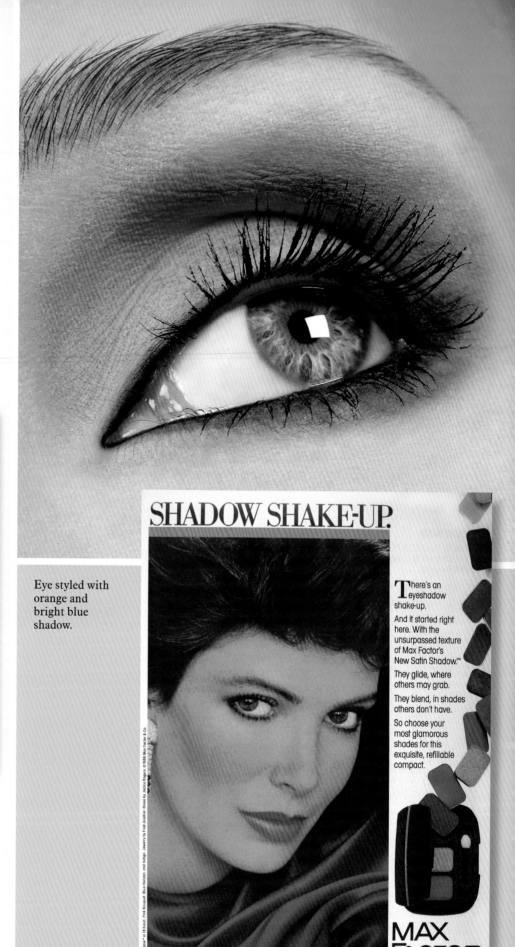

Eye styled with orange and bright blue shadow.

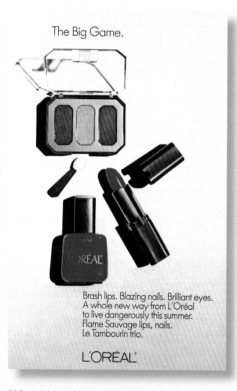

The Big Game.

Brash lips. Blazing nails. Brilliant eyes. A whole new way from L'Oréal to live dangerously this summer. Flame Sauvage lips, nails. Le Tambourin trio.

L'ORÉAL

L'Oréal brand cosmetics in vibrant colors advertisement, c. 1980s.

Max Factor brand Satin Shadow advertisement, 1986.

SHADOW SHAKE-UP.

There's an eyeshadow shake-up.

And it started right here. With the unsurpassed texture of Max Factor's New Satin Shadow.™

They glide, where others may grab.

They blend, in shades others don't have.

So choose your most glamorous shades for this exquisite, refillable compact.

MAX FACTOR

MAKES YOUR BEAUTY COME TO LIFE

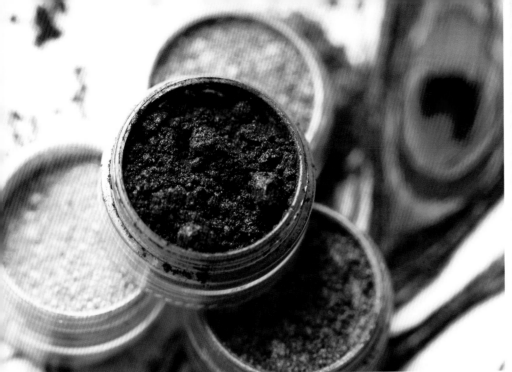

Lips

Lips are lined using a fuchsia or dark red liner slightly exaggerated and filled in with fuchsia or red lipstick.

Powder shadows in bright peacock feather hues.

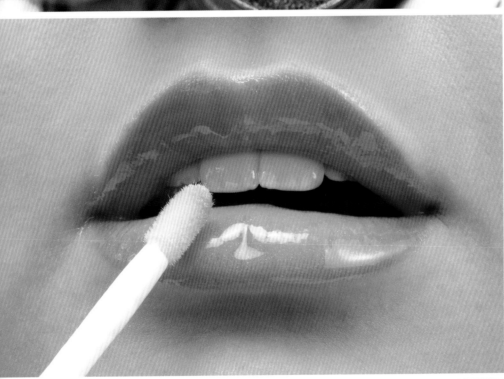

Lips with pink-tinted gloss.

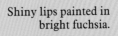
Shiny lips painted in bright fuchsia.

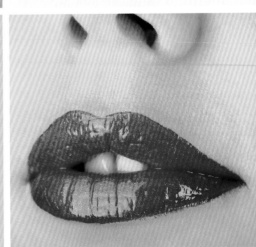

173

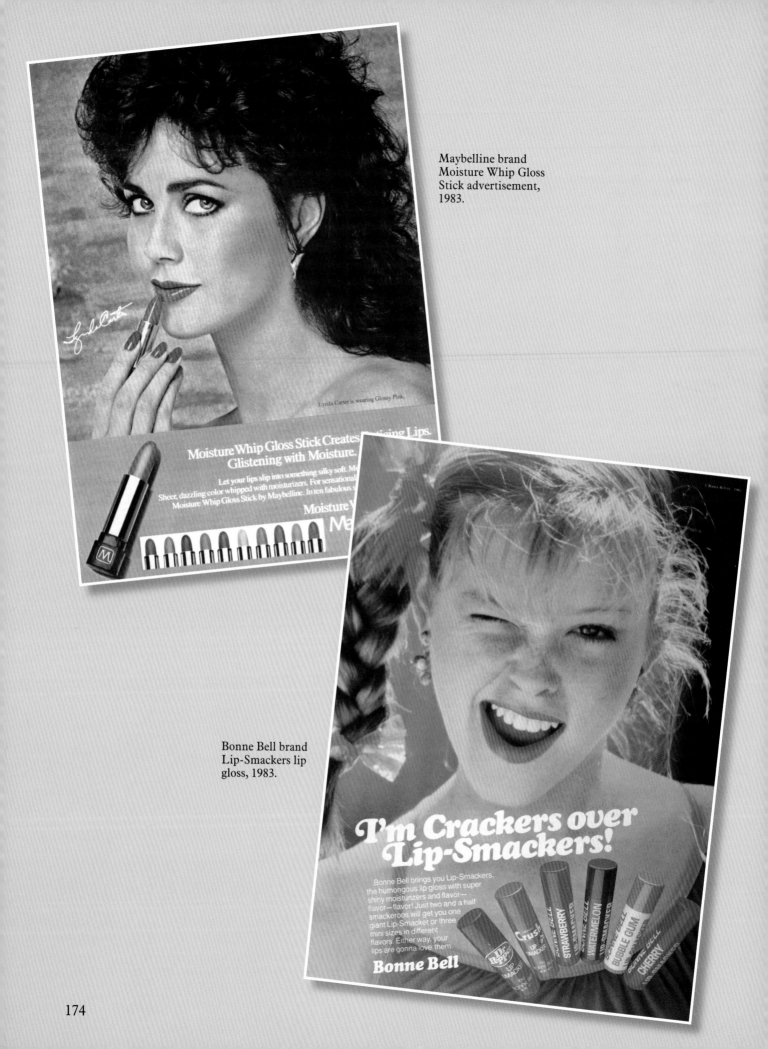

Maybelline brand
Moisture Whip Gloss
Stick advertisement,
1983.

Bonne Bell brand
Lip-Smackers lip
gloss, 1983.

174

Nails

Nails are long and bright, and painted with bright reds, oranges, and fuchsias.

Natural nails with a longer length in a French-style become popular at the end of the decade.

Revlon brand nail colors advertisement, 1984.

Maybelline brand Pearliest ManiCure Nail Color advertisement, c. 1984.

175

The 1990s

Modern depiction of 1990s style makeup.

America was in a state of worry. The media's focus was on issues such as the AIDS epidemic, unemployment, and the turmoil in the Middle East. Crisis brought on a time for change and new leadership as baby boomer Bill Clinton was elected president of the United States. The stock market and economy flourished. But Clinton's second term in office was punctuated with an infidelity scandal and the threat of impeachment. At the end of the decade, the country went back to a conservative leadership base as George W. Bush was elected president in 2000. Continued development of the Internet connected the globe at lightning speed. Cellular phones and laptop computers were readily available and affordable to the average citizen. Businesses around the world shifted from "bricks to clicks," and the virtual office replaced the setting of Melanie Griffith's *Working Girl* a decade earlier.

Because people were busier than ever, eating right became a challenge. PowerBars and other meal choices flooded the market shelves to meet the demands of always on-the-go consumers. Globalization, made possible by increased communication through the internet, made a wide variety of products virtually available to anyone anywhere. The rise and popularity of coffeehouse chains such as Starbucks and The Coffee Bean & Tea Leaf became an alternative office and meeting place, offering more personal freedom from the dreaded cramped cubicles and staunch offices of corporate America.

A shift from the corporate looks of the 1980s led to a more relaxed work environment that created a more casual, less rigid look. A comfortable, informal attitude toward fashion was deemed acceptable. "Casual Friday," the day when employees were permitted to dress down, was introduced throughout companies across the country. Clothing stores such as The Gap emerged with generic urban clothes—clean, neutral cottons, jeans, and t-shirts— suitable for everyday wear. Designers stepped up to the demand for easier, wearable fabrics with a casual but luxurious feel, notably with the use of Tencel, and an upscale look that would allow women to go from work to play.

Victoria's Secret lingerie stores gained popularity when the company began using supermodels such as Naomi Campbell, Stephanie Seymour, and Claudia Schiffer in its advertising campaigns and fashion shows. Like the Madonna-driven trend of underwear as outerwear of the 1980s, the look continued throughout the 1990s. Undergarments were often visible under suit jackets and sheer clothing. The trend of voluptuous breasts was popularized by Victoria's Secret's padded, boosting Wonderbra for women who wanted an ample bosom without the cost of augmentation surgery.

The world of fashion was highly eclectic. Major trends included waist-high denim jeans, tight leotard bodysuits worn under boxy trousers, baby doll dresses, and baggy overalls. Women in their teens through twenties embraced retro styles inspired by the big band swing movement of the 1940s. The grunge look of torn jeans, flannel shirts, and worker boots was a trend that would be forever tied to the decade. Thrift shops and army surplus stores became common places for the youth culture to attain their wardrobes. Adolescents adopted loose cargo pants and fitness sportswear as a general uniform.

Toward the end of the 1980s, makeup trends followed the neutral tones and practical styles associated with the yuppies, or young urban professionals. Wearing strong makeup was considered out of style, and the face was natural looking as women embraced a sleek, minimalist, no makeup look. Showing off well cared for skin became a status symbol. With hydrated skin and glossy lips, a subtly painted face was considered in. Continuing into the decade, women wore earthy tones, bronzer with eyeliner and opted for a nude matte lipstick. Some gloss was worn to enhance the natural beauty of the full lips. Women re-discovered the charm of the old-fashioned styles, bringing a resurgence of retro packaging and smaller niche brands. Brands from the past such as Creed perfume and LeClerc powder, both from the late 1800s, were reintroduced to the market. Prescriptives, a custom blended makeup line, provided women with a personal shopping experience.

Hairstyles were kept simple. Bobs and long, straight hair were popular using hair bands to pull back and emphasize the shape of the face. The only similarity to the glitter usage during the 1980s, was a subtle, but new iridescent shimmer used in makeup and hair spray. The full-bodied, chin-length haircut that was popularized by Jennifer Aniston, and the funkier choppier hairstyle of Meg Ryan were the decade's defining hair trends. Hair extensions and a wide variety of hair colors opened the field of hairstyles to experimentation and the usage of more unique hair colors.

The alternative music world brought on the grungy look of smeared makeup and dirty, unkempt hair. Body decorations such as tattoos and henna became popular ways to adorn the body. Brands began to offer decorative decals to place on the skin. Multiple body piercings, through the ears, tongue, navel, and eyebrows, were also in vogue. Social gatherings known as raves became a new way for young people to gather and express themselves freely and creatively. Ravers entranced themselves with hallucinogenic drugs and techno music.

Peeling and dermabrasion treatments became more mainstream. Injection of collagen was used to fill in lines and smooth out wrinkles. Consumers believed in the "right to be young" or to look as young as one felt. Water-based products such as bottle water, designer water, and bars that offered expensive brand name water, rose in consumption. Mineral water brand Evian tied its pink-labeled bottles to being healthy and beautiful inside and out. Beauty spas throughout the country grew in popularity going from thirty in 1990 to six hundred by 1999. Hotels joined this trend by offering in-house spa services to their guests.

The battle to rid the body of cellulite with expensive creams and body-toners dominated the market, while a growing interest in celebrity looks saw top makeup artists such as Bobbi Brown launch highly successful independent cosmetic lines.

Since women realized more and more that health and beauty were attributed to taking care of one's inside as well as one's outside, fitness trends in food and exercise became daily rituals. Body massages and holistic treatments were equally as important as a healthy diet. Strength and spiritual workouts such as yoga and Pilates replaced aerobics and jogging as the hottest trends in the fitness world.

Kate Moss embodied the new "heroin chic" look of very slim androgynous models. Supermodel Iman, frustrated by the appalling lack of ranges in makeup shades to suit women of color, succeeded with her own makeup line. Meanwhile, Isabella Rossellini, famously dropped by Lancome at 43 for being too old, launched her own Manifesto range, designed for women of all ages. Actresses replaced supermodels as spokespeople for cosmetic companies, since it was found that women could identify with closer to normal-sized actresses more than with the six-foot, 90-pound, size zero unattainable figures associated with a supermodel.

Decade Highlights

- President George Bush deploys U.S. troops to Saudi Arabia for Operation Desert Shield in 1990.
- Texture is introduced to nail designs. Montage nails with hologram and quartz are popular styles.
- The short, square, white-tipped French manicure is the predominant look of nails.
- Catherine Deneuve represents YSL's Prelude a la Beaute line.
- French makeup artist Laura Mercier starts a cosmetics line in 1996 that bears her name. She becomes widely known for her VHS tape called "The Flawless Finish."
- Clinique sells 14 million bottles of foundation per year, with its best selling formula being Balanced Makeup.
- Chanel's "Les Contrastes" plays light and dark shades off of each other. A matte face accentuates bright lips and dark, smoldering eyes.
- Shiseido's Eau de Soin is a fragrance that is said to relax and energize.
- Prescriptives introduces Exact Color, a "minimalist" approach, to color based on basic skin-tone groups.
- Shiseido introduces Les Suprematistes, with a philosophy to reduce makeup colors to simple triads.
- Paris image creator Serge Lutens chooses the colors red, black, and white to paint a subtle face.
- The "squoval" shape is born in the fall of '93. For shorter nails, square and oval are mixed for a delicate and feminine look.
- Acrylic overlays with French tips, as well as appliqué gold charms, are all the rage during the summer of '95.
- Makeup artist Alexis Vogel establishes her own signature makeup line and "system" and is credited with creating Pamela Anderson's "sex kitten" look.
- "In the '80s it was so incredibly over the top. Now it's about how we can express ourselves and still maintain a certain amount of dignity." Isaac Mizrahi

The Face

Eyebrows are of a medium thickness and groomed.

Smoky, neutral shades with liquid liner are used around the eye.

Matte foundations one shade lighter than one's skin tone is applied for a porcelain look.

Matte reds and wine lipstick shades are used for evening, and metallic neutrals with lips lined with a lip pencil are used for day.

Soft blush is added to the apples of the cheeks for a healthy glow along with a color-coordinating lipstick.

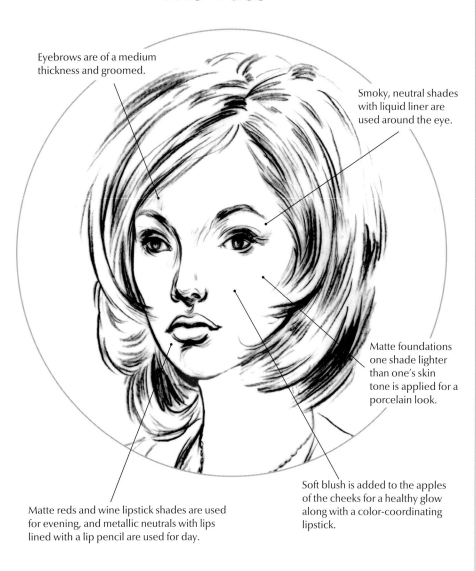

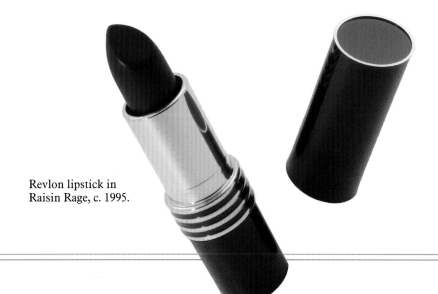

Revlon lipstick in Raisin Rage, c. 1995.

COLOR PALETTE
of the
1990s

LIQUID OR CREAM

Porcelain Flesh   Honey   Tan

POWDER

Shimmer / Translucent

BLUSH

Light Rose   Light Coral

SHADOW

Maroon   Purple   Orange

 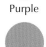

Camel   Gray   Teak

MASCARA   LINER

Burgundy   Brown   Black

LIPSTICK

Smoky Rose   Red Brick   Matte Nude   Berry

Scarlet   Plum Brown   Nude Frost   Russet

The 1990s Face
Makeup Becomes Efficient

The neutral look of makeup prevails even though women are using more makeup to create a polished and well-defined face. The matte porcelain face is the perfect foundation to emphasize the lips and eyes.

Consumers become increasingly sophisticated. A desire to enhance one's natural beauty with lighter, less visible formulas results in a scientific approach to cosmetics. Research and development of new technologies and new ingredients becomes the major push for larger brands. Cosmetics no longer just cover-up, but are also "light-reflecting" and "wrinkle-defying."

Companies add anti-aging ingredients to makeup. Vitamin A acid and retinol are popular choices found in many products on the market. AHA fruit acids are used in formulations by the Estée Lauder company.

Cosmetic companies advertise their products as being "intelligent" and are able to determine where the skin needs more or less moisture or nutrients.

The decade sees an explosion of makeup products in the market, making cosmetics accessible to more women. With less time to dedicate to their image, makeup is more practical and easy to apply.

Skin is very tanned, two tones above the skin's natural color. Long sunbathing sessions outdoors or in tanning salons are common.

Skin with glitter or brilliant powders on cleavage is all the rage. A liner is used two tones above the lips' color.

Eyebrows are groomed to be naturally shaped and not too thin. They tend to point upward to a point.

Eyes are lifted and lengthened with shading.

Neutral-colored rouge is packaged in color-coordinated combination packs.

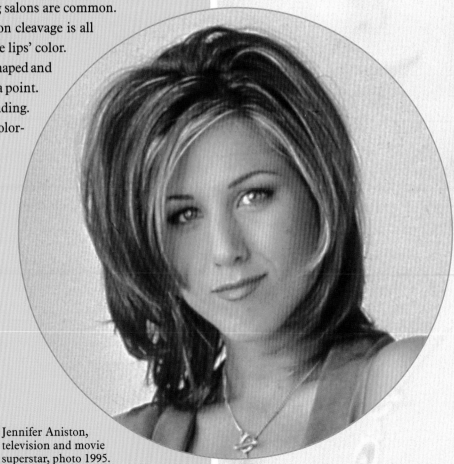

Jennifer Aniston, television and movie superstar, photo 1995.

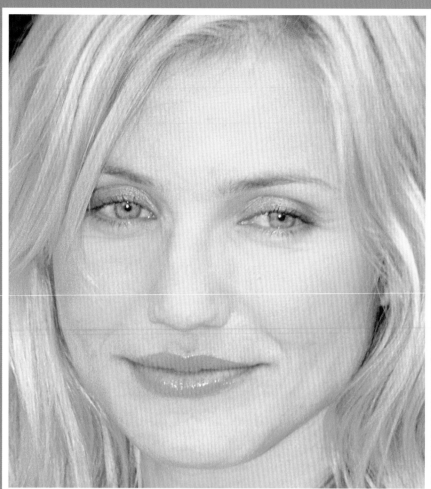

Cameron Diaz, Hollywood actress, photo c. late 1990s.

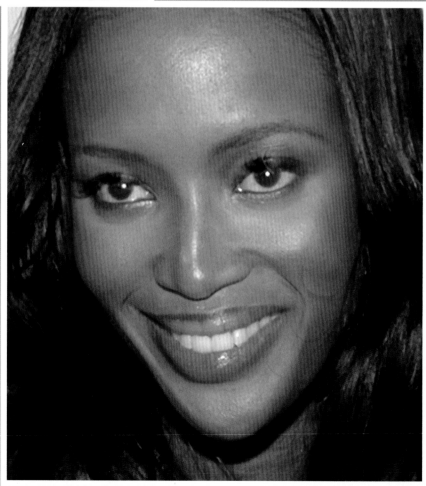

Naomi Campbell, British supermodel, photo c. late 1990s.

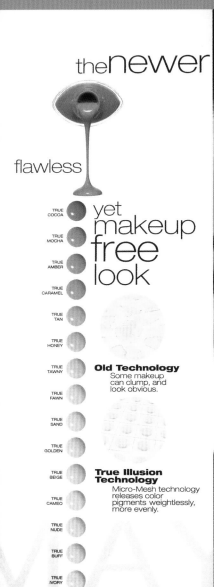

the newer natural

flawless

yet makeup free look

TRUE COCOA	
TRUE MOCHA	
TRUE AMBER	
TRUE CARAMEL	
TRUE TAN	
TRUE HONEY	
TRUE TAWNY	**Old Technology** Some makeup can clump, and look obvious.
TRUE FAWN	
TRUE SAND	
TRUE GOLDEN	
TRUE BEIGE	**True Illusion Technology** Micro-Mesh technology releases color pigments weightlessly, more evenly.
TRUE CAMEO	
TRUE NUDE	
TRUE BUFF	
TRUE IVORY	

©1999 Maybelline Inc.
Tomiko is wearing True Illusion Makeup and True Illusion Pressed Powder in True Cocoa.

Maybelline brand True Illusion Makeup and True Illusion Pressed Powder advertisement, 1999.

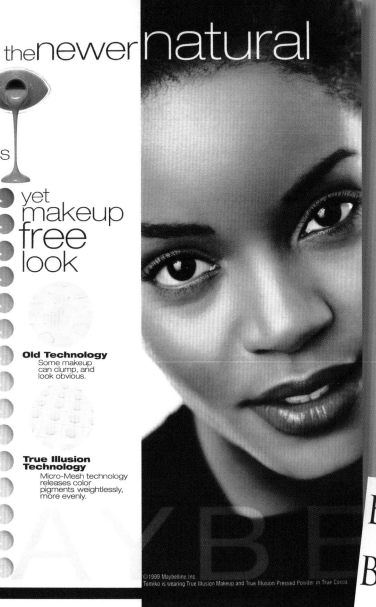

Actress Salma Hayek, May 18, 2008.

Foundation

Lighter face foundations are announced monthly and by the end of the decade there are many types in the marketplace.

Foundations used are typically of a matte, porcelain finish in a shade lighter than one's skin tone.

Liquid or cream foundation is applied all over the face and topped with a dusting of powder.

Cream foundation is also used on the eyelids in place of eye shadow or eyeliners for a no makeup look.

Neutrogena brand Healthy Skin Liquid Makeup advertisement, 1999.

Blush

Cheeks are shaded in the same color as lips.

A new product called a liquid-to-powder blush is dotted along the cheekbone. It dries to a light, powder finish to give a soft, natural look.

The apples of the cheeks wear minimal color with just a touch of blush for a healthy glow.

The prominent blush shades are creamy pink, dusty rose, and neutral or bronze.

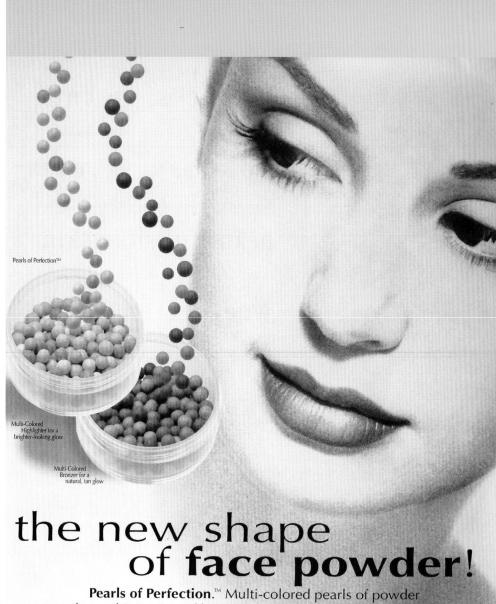

Pearls of Perfection™

Multi-Colored Highlighter for a brighter-looking glow

Multi-Colored Bronzer for a natural, tan glow

the new shape of **face powder!**

Pearls of Perfection.™ Multi-colored pearls of powder capture the sophistication of loose powder without the mess. Now, you can keep it loose and keep it together! Just the right combination of colors is brought together to naturally enhance your skin tone with a subtle glow. Brush it on and let loose the power of pearls!

PHYSICIANS FORMULA®

Hypoallergenic Corrective Cosmetics

© Pierre Fabre, Inc. 1999

Consumer Help Line 1 800 227 0333, www.PhysiciansFormula.com, At fine Drug and Discount Stores everywhere!

Physicians Formula brand Pearls of Perfection powder advertisement, 1999.

Eyes

Mysterious eyes in smoky, earthy shades are created to enhance a woman's features without looking overdone.

The most typical '90s shading is a horizontal, U-shaped gradient effect that slightly emphasizes the eye socket.

The outer third part of the eye's inner line is defined.

Black, brown, transparent, and even blue and green mascaras are worn. Shadows feature earth tones that are deepened by various intensities of black eye shadow liner. Shadows are muted, but the eye receives more emphasis with liquid eyeliner around the entire eye.

A hint of bold color such as orange, burgundy, or purple is blended with smoky charcoal on the eye.

A light shade is applied on the lid, a darker shade in the crease, and a highlighter on the brow bone.

A bit of pencil in the far corners and burgundy mascara add drama for an evening look.

Eye colors in monochromatic shades such as gray, bisque, camel, smoke, and muted blues and greens are offered with a hint of shine.

Eye pencils are used to achieve a softer, more contoured effect. They come in earthen tones such as camel, granite, and brown.

Eyebrows are of medium thickness and groomed, since a sportier look is popular.

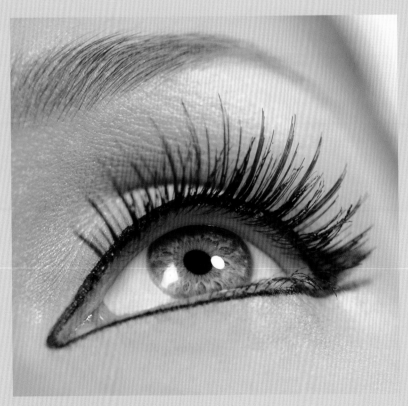

Eye with false eyelashes, painted with shadow and lined entirely with eyeliner.

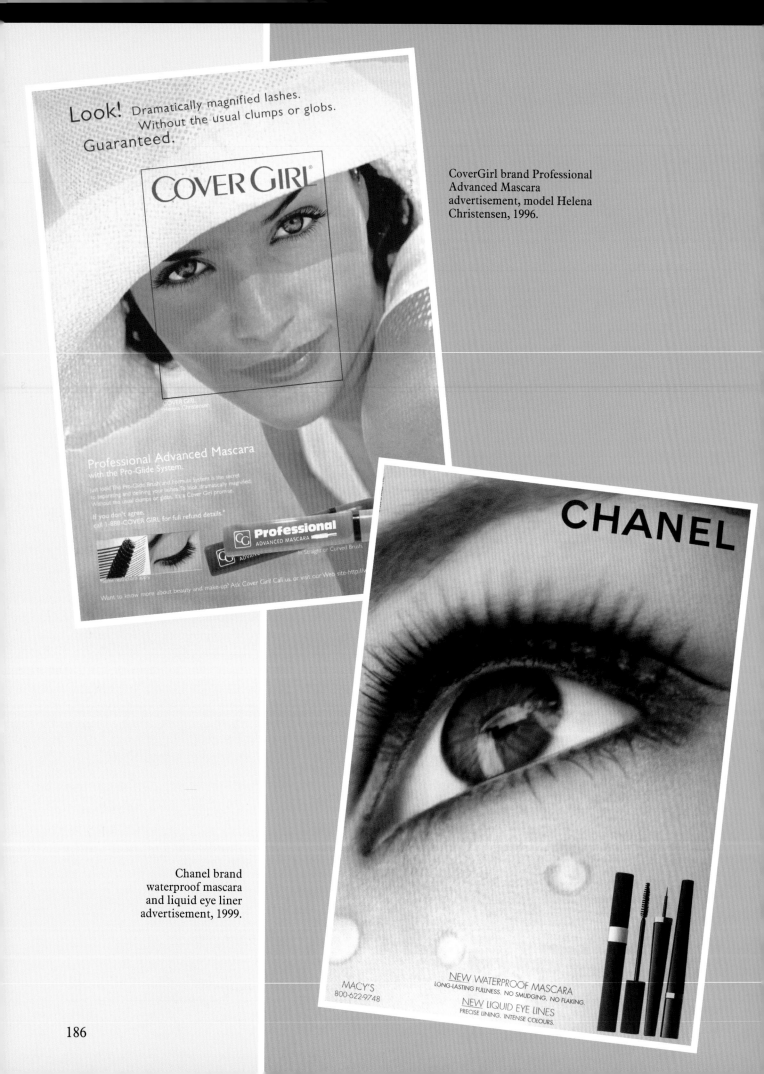

Look! Dramatically magnified lashes. Without the usual clumps or globs. Guaranteed.

COVER GIRL®

Professional Advanced Mascara
with the Pro-Glide System.

CoverGirl brand Professional Advanced Mascara advertisement, model Helena Christensen, 1996.

CHANEL

Chanel brand waterproof mascara and liquid eye liner advertisement, 1999.

MACY'S
800-622-9748

NEW WATERPROOF MASCARA
LONG-LASTING FULLNESS. NO SMUDGING. NO FLAKING.

NEW LIQUID EYE LINES
PRECISE LINING. INTENSE COLOURS.

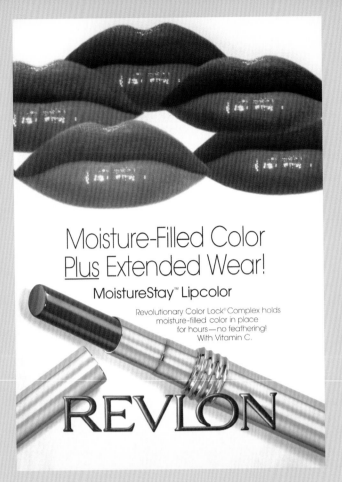

Revlon brand MoistureStay™ Lipcolor advertisement, 1999.

Lips

New lip colors involve vibrant shades of matte red, plums, and satin reds. Women use pencil techniques to achieve full, plump lips, or to shape imperfect lips.

Deep red wine-colored lipsticks and lip liners are used for an evening look, while daytime lipstick colors include light browns, neutrals, and pink hues with liners.

Lip liners are worn without lipstick or gloss.

Also popular are bright colors with shades in scarlet, blued berries, burnt reds, russets, and neutrals with metallic accents.

Lip coloring pencils finish the look.

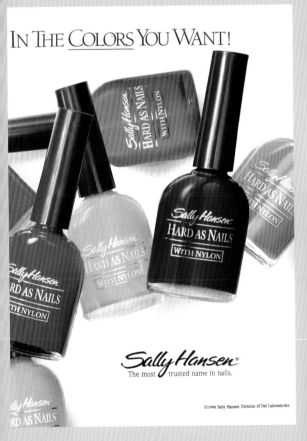

Sally Hansen brand Hard As Nails nail polish advertisement, 1996.

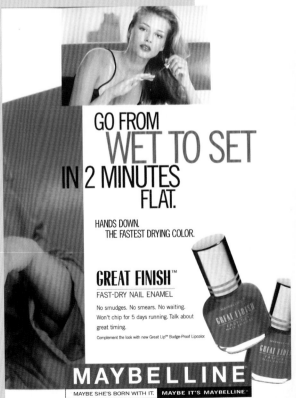

Maybelline brand Great Finish Fast-Dry Nail Enamel advertisement, 1996.

Nails

Cosmetic companies let go of the idea of matching lip and nail colors and start producing blue, green, and a host of other exotic colors such as gold, silver, black, and neon.

Artificial nails become a popular trend as nails reach longer lengths.

The 2000s

Modern depiction of 2000s style makeup.

The millennium brought on vast advancements in the field of communications. Information was delivered at optimum speeds through the World Wide Web. Since the news was concurrently updated online, the decade saw a decline in print media as daily papers reported yesterday's news. Public opinion reigned supreme as people posted comments on blogs, message boards, and chat rooms. The Internet became a launching tool for those seeking job opportunities, soul mates, or an online education. Businesses experienced a "dot com" revolution as web-based conferencing, online banking, and stock trading sites made performing transactions convenient and economically time saving.

The stock market crashed in April of 2000. Many of the risky start-up and dot com businesses lost all of their value at once. The few web-based companies who managed to survive and grow established their marks as Internet success stories. Among them were Jerry Yang of Yahoo! and Jeff Bezos of Amazon.com.

The dominating presence of the non-scripted "reality" show became a prominent genre in television. Competition shows such as *Survivor*, *American Idol*, and *The Amazing Race* proved to be top ratings winners and created instant celebrities out of average American citizens. Shows such as *Extreme Makeover* and *The Biggest Loser* inspired viewers to enhance their outward appearance, whether it was through plastic surgery or exercise.

As the first decade of the new millennium moved on, the Great Recession devastated the mortgage business, the economy, and the future of millions of American families. The economy was riddled with unemployment, financial instability, and the collapse of the housing market. Consumers turned to big-box retailers such as Target and Walmart and warehouse membership stores such as Costco and Sam's Club. These discount stores offered shoppers high quality generic brands and brand name merchandise at affordable prices.

With an increased awareness of global climate change and a push toward all things environmental, a trend toward organically and locally grown protein and produce became evident during the decade. Consumers were knowledgeable as to what they put in their bodies and how products came to their table. Americans continued their obsession with dieting as counting calories shifted to a consciousness of the intake of fat, then to sugar, then to carbohydrates, then back to calories.

Fashion and pop culture became tied more than ever. Celebrities such as Victoria Beckham, Gwen Stefani, Kim Kardashian, and Jennifer Lopez released their own clothing lines hoping to lure trend-seeking consumers attracted by their fame. Celebutante Paris Hilton brought back an updated version of the blond bombshell with her glossy pink lips and platinum blond hair. Singer-songwriter Amy Winehouse's beehive hairdos and thick-winged eyeliner inspired a short-lived fashion following reminiscent of the girl groups of the 1960s.

The grunge movement of the 1990s came to a close and led to the introduction of more revealing fashion trends. Low-rise and tight jeans, dark leggings, and velour track suits were dominating fashion trends. By mid-decade, fashion was a hodgepodge of styles as it was influenced by the preppy, hippie, and Bohemian looks of the 1950s and '60s. These mass-marketed clothing trends were found at such retail chains as Old Navy, The Gap, and Banana Republic.

The hip hop movement was the source of a trend in urban wear for men. Oversized shirts and baggy pants worn well below the waistline, backward-facing baseball caps, and sports sneakers defined the "ghetto fabulous" look. In general, collared polo shirts and buttoned short sleeved shirts were worn untucked from pants. The decade also saw the introduction of the metrosexual male. Celebrities like Kanye West and athlete David Beckham showed men that it was okay to take care of their looks with products most commonly associated with beauty-conscious females. Several cosmetic lines entered the market with male grooming products.

Permanent body art such as tattoos and more adventurous body piercings continued to be popular with adolescents and adults in their twenties and thirties. The South Asian forehead decoration known as a bindi and henna tattooing worn by Madonna were hot trends throughout the decade. Skin jewelry took the form of self adhesive crystals arranged in patterns. Crystals and fake gems were also added to manicured nails.

From the beginning to the middle of the decade, celebrities inspired a no-makeup look. Often seen on the red carpet, actresses wore bare faces evened out with tinted moisturizer and glowing shimmer highlights. Subtle color stains on the cheeks added to a dewy, natural look. Face and body bronzers were the perfect accompaniment to this luminous look.

Other trends for the decade included budget luxury cosmetics or high quality cosmetics at over-the-counter prices, do-it-yourself salon services such as kits for at home manicures, pedicures, waxes and dermabrasions, and beauty products as fashion accessories such as costume jewelry that held lip gloss and solid perfume.

Botox and other injectibles used as wrinkle reducers became the most popular cosmetic drug in the world. Women held Botox parties where guests sipped cocktails and received botox injections as well as other spa treatments.

As the first decade of the millennium came to a close, the processed tan and sparkle look subsided toward a more natural look in makeup. Continuing into the next decade of the millennium, beauty brands turned to functional, beneficial makeup. The cosmeceutical began entering the market, combining the fashion aspects of color with the benefits of skincare.

Decade Highlights

- The staying power of lipsticks improves with the release of Maybelline's line of Superstay lipstick in 2005.
- Clinique releases 'stay the day' color.
- New all-in-one facial and toning cleansers replace separate cleansers and toners.
- Throw away cleanser wipes made by L'Oréal Plenitude, Nivea, and Oil of Olay remove both eye makeup and lipstick gently.
- Aromatherapy products for face, body, and hair take on a huge percentage of the market as self indulgent pampering becomes the norm. High end products include Decleor's Aromessence with neroli oil, Elemis milk bath, L'Occitane's pure soap products, and Jo Malone's bath essences.
- Consumers become very aware of skin cancer. Makeup bronzing products are improved to give consumers a naturally tanned look without the sun or use of a tanning salon.
- Kevyn Aucoin emerges as a top makeup artist, releasing several books and his own makeup line. He works as a makeup artist from the age of twenty-one until his death at age forty in May of 2002.
- The makers of Botox introduce Latisse, a topical solution that grows one's eye lashes.

The Face

Shimmer in pink creams or liquid stains in rosy shades are applied on the apples of the cheeks and tops of cheekbones.

Eyebrows are shaped professionally with a high arch that lifts the eye upward.

Eye shadows in light or neutral and darker pastels are applied.

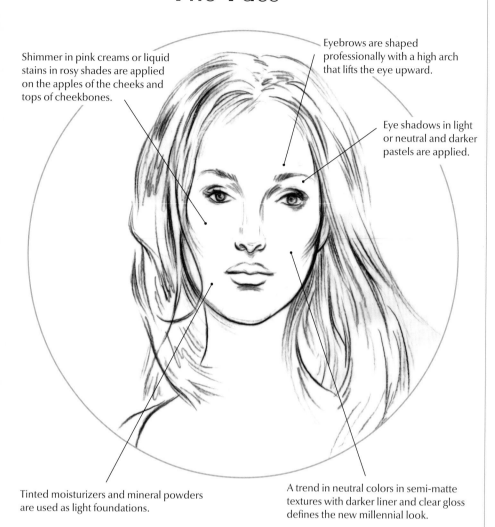

Tinted moisturizers and mineral powders are used as light foundations.

A trend in neutral colors in semi-matte textures with darker liner and clear gloss defines the new millennial look.

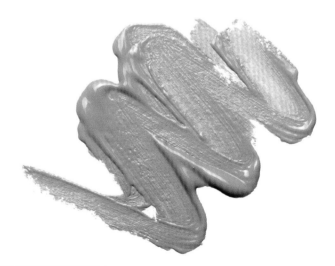

COLOR PALETTE of the 2000s

LIGHT LIQUID / POWDER

Flesh   Translucent

BLUSH

Warm Soft Blush   Rose

SHADOW

Lilac   Chestnut Brown   Soft Pink

Purple Frost   Taupe   Slate Gray

LINER

Black   Indigo

LIPSTICK

Warm Pink   Light Chocolate   Nude

Pink Frost   Reddish Brown   Natural Pink   Pale Mauve

The 2000s Face
Pop Culture Looks

The first decade of the new millennium sees a usage in gel eyeliners that are longer-wearing and easier to apply than liquid liners.

New powder, gel, and liquid makeup formulas create many variations in makeup finishes such as matte, semi-matte, and dewy.

Nude colors are in for day looks. Deep, bright colors are in for evening looks.

Makeup is very wearable for most women, since there are so many looks available from sheer and natural to all out glam.

A 1940s-inspired look takes on a modern twist. Red wine lips, soft black or gray eyeliner on top lashes, a soft rosy cheek, and a light eye shadow define this retro look.

Light chestnut brown in the crease of the eye, warm brown as a contour under the cheekbone, and a nude glossy lip creates the perfect modern face for day.

Although mineral-based cosmetics are introduced in the 1970s, its usage gains popularity in the 2000s. Mineral cosmetic brands such as Bare Escentuals and Sheer Cover create powder makeup that offers just as much coverage as a liquid foundation, but is much gentler on the skin.

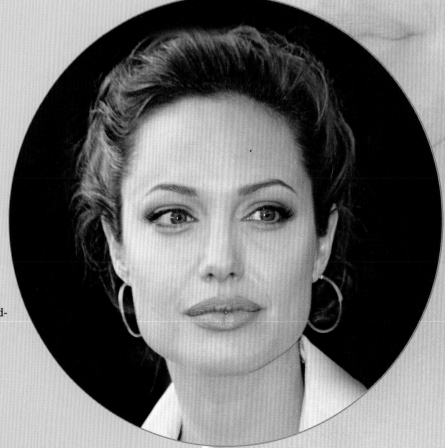

Angelina Jolie, award-winning actress and humanitarian, photo 2004.

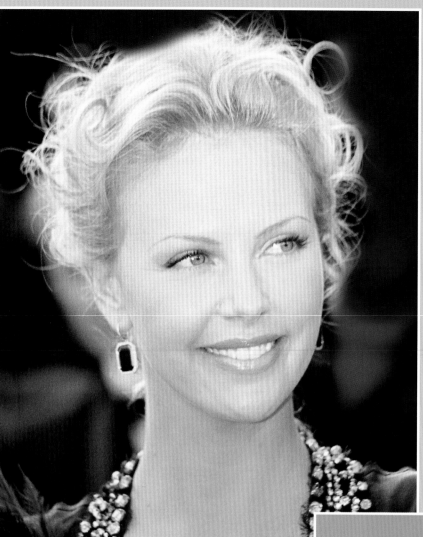

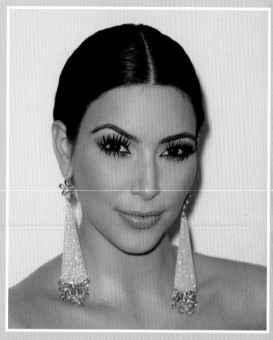

Charlize Theron, international screen star, photo 2004.

Kim Kardashian, model and personality, 2011.

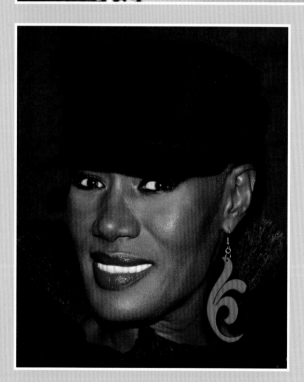

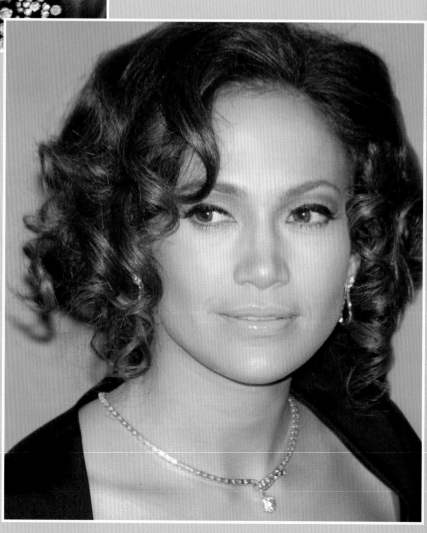

Grace Jones, actress and model, was the original face of MAC cosmetics. Today, women of color including Queen Latifah, Sofia Vergara, Eva Longoria, and Jennifer Lopez are used to promote mainstream cosmetics brands like L'Oreal and Cover Girl to an increasingly diverse global market.

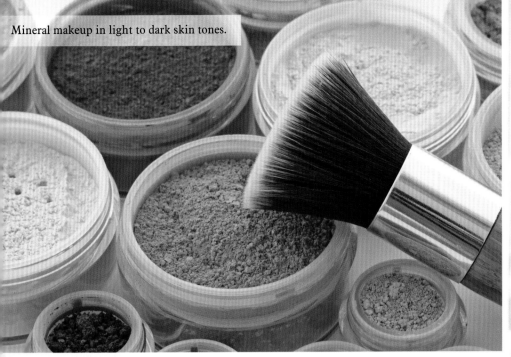

Mineral makeup in light to dark skin tones.

Foundation

A sheer primer on the face, with cream concealer is used to hide skin imperfections.

For flawless looking skin with a slightly matte finish, a liquid foundation is used to cover every imperfection.

Tinted moisturizer with silicone contains ingredients that would stand up to heat and humidity and provides light to medium coverage. New formulas contain SPF with long lasting wear and an invisible feel.

Cream foundation is used for a natural or nude look.

L'Oréal brand Visible Lift Line Minimizing Makeup advertisement, model Andie MacDowell, 2003.

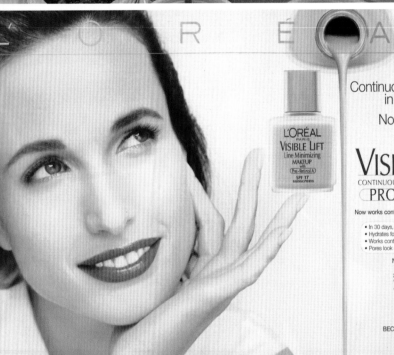

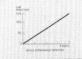

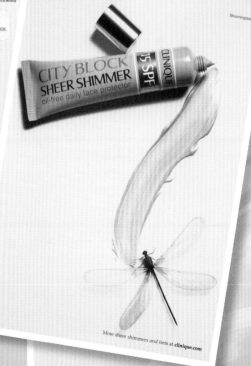

Clinique brand City Block Sheer Shimmer face protector advertisement, 2003.

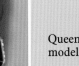

Queen Latifah, actress and model, Hollywood, CA, 2009.

Blush

Cheeks shimmer with less color and more glow.

Subtle color in a soft white, cream, or pink shimmer is applied to the apples of the cheeks, or onto the top of the cheekbones.

Shimmer sticks in tubes similar to twist up lipstick tubes, or even shimmer eye shadows are used on the cheeks.

Bright, rosy red tints and stains are used to color the cheeks.

Warm brown is used for contouring under the cheekbones.

To minimize a chiseled look of high cheekbones, a soft blush is added to the lower cheeks and sides of nose.

Maybelline brand shimmery cosmetics advertisement, model Josie Maran, 2003.

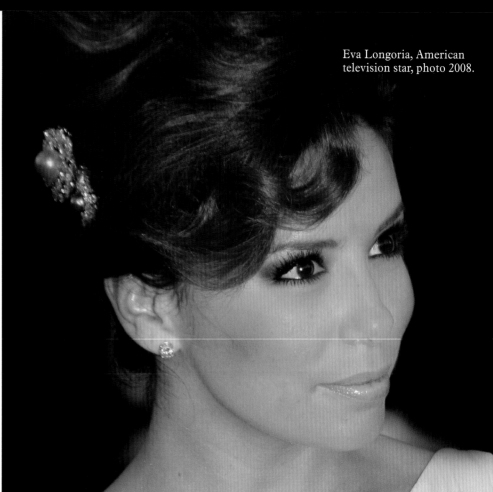

Eva Longoria, American television star, photo 2008.

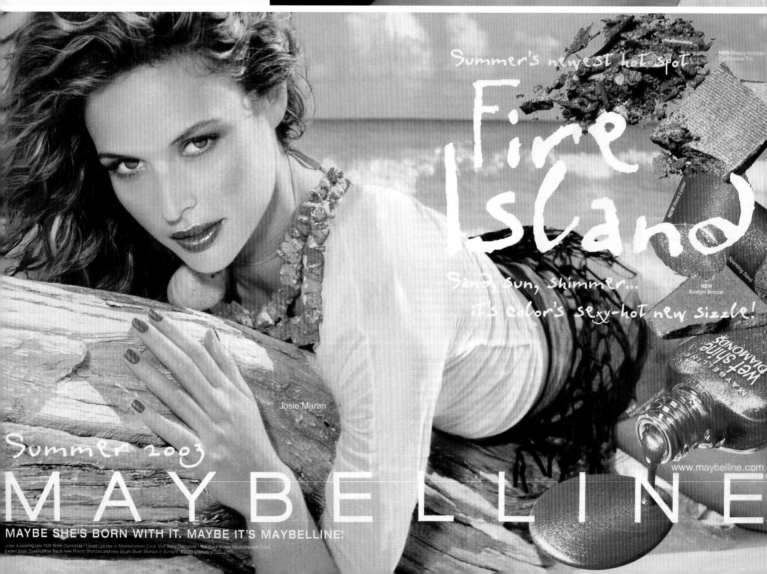

Summer's newest hot spot

Fire Island

Sand, sun, shimmer...
it's color's sexy-hot new sizzle!

Josie Maran

Summer 2003

www.maybelline.com

MAYBELLINE

MAYBE SHE'S BORN WITH IT. MAYBE IT'S MAYBELLINE.

Eyes

Soft pinks, blues, greens, and lilacs are on the decade's color palette for a sheer water-color effect.

Sheers are applied around the entire eye, both under lashes and on the eyelid. A coat of mascara on the top and bottom lashes finishes off the look.

A sheer, shimmery, sparkly white is applied either on the lid, on the eye brow bone, or over the whole eye. The look takes on a shimmery ice crystal quality.

A light colored luminescent shadow or highlighter covers the upper part of the eyelid to the eyebrow.

A darker pastel shade is used on the eyelid fold along with a dark glossy shade on the lower edge to the lashes.

Very thin black eyeliner and black mascara is used for a dramatic long lash look.

On the inner edge of the lash, a thin white "kajal" pencil is used to make the eyes appear brighter.

Professional eyebrow shaping lifts, contours, and frames the face. It gives an instant effect of a mini face lift and involves waxing and plucking of the brow hairs for a precise outline.

The eastern method of threading is considered to be the most superior way of removing brow hair.

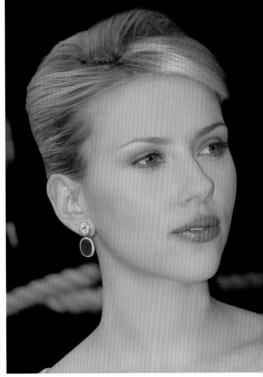

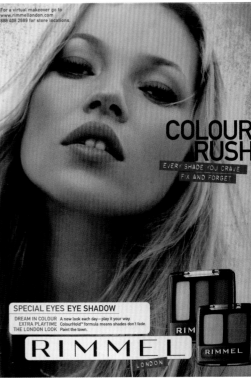

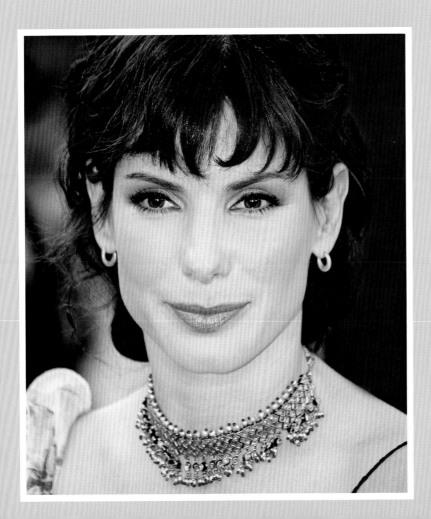

Top:
Scarlett Johansson, American motion picture actress, photo 2005.

Above:
Rimmel brand eye shadow advertisement, model Kate Moss, 2005.

Left:
Sandra Bullock, award-winning screen star, photo 2002.

197

Lips

Reddish-brown reds or close-to-natural shade lip color in semi-gloss is used. The color is applied by drawing the outline and filling in the color using a brush for a clean shape.

A darker liner is worn with a lighter shade of lipstick.

Clear lip gloss is used for a clean daytime look.

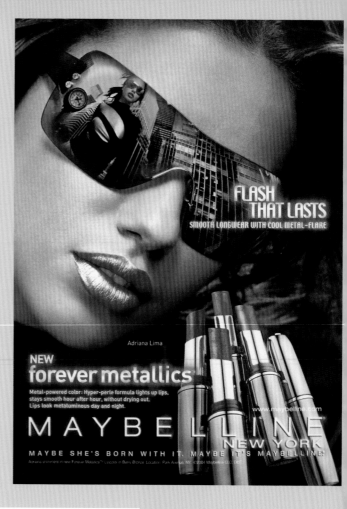

Maybelline brand Forever Metallics lipstick advertisement, model Adriana Lima, 2001.

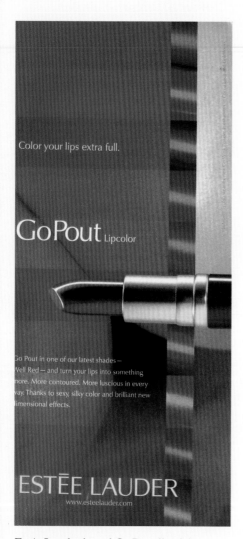

Estée Lauder brand Go Pout lipstick advertisement, 2000.

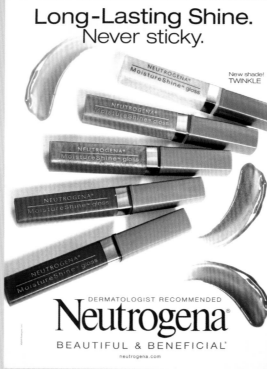

Neutrogena brand MoistureShine gloss lip gloss advertisement, 2004.

Olay brand ColorMoist Lipstick advertisement, 2000.

198

Nails

The early 2000s gives way to a back-to-natural look. Nails are delicate and feminine in appearance, showing off a natural, well-kept look.

The reverse French manicure with clear tips is popular with brides in the summer of 2001.

Short, natural, and polished nails are all the rage with colorful nail polishes that offer a quick dose of style. Dark nail polish enters mainstream use with the introduction of Black Satin nail polish by Chanel. Other dark colors such as navy, chocolate brown, forest green, and dark purple are seen on everyone from trendy teens to business professionals.

Metallics and vivid colors are worn for day and night.

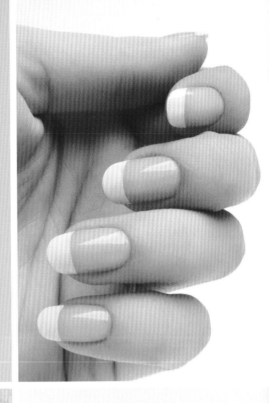

French-manicured fingernail tips—known as the classic "pink and white."

In 2010, CND Creative Nail Design introduced Shellac, a hybrid acrylic-type nail enhancement that could be applied like polish. Light-cured gel nails followed.

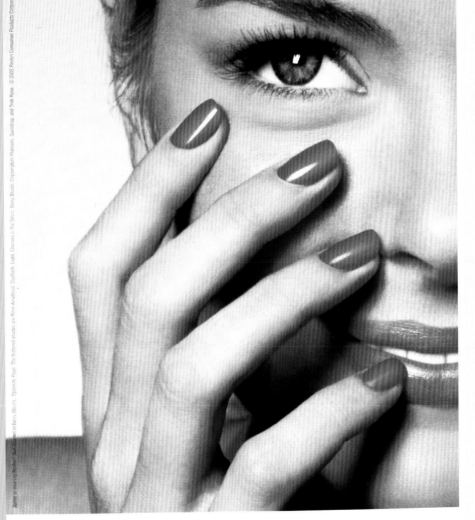

Revlon brand nail enamel advertisement, 2003.

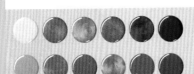

Product Development
TIMELINE
3000 B.C. to A.D. 1558

3000 B.C.
Women of the Orient use a powder called batikka made from powdered marble, rice, and borax.

2200 B.C.
Assyrians' early recipes for hair dyes are made from cassia and leek extract. Mineral-colored paste paints the eyes. Green is the most predominant color.

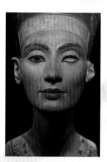

1300 B.C.
The toilette box of the Egyptian woman Thuthu, wife of scribe Ani, contains pumice stones, eye paints of mineral powders and applicators, liquid colors in small containers, and palettes for mixing any shade needed. Professional stylists are employed by wealthy women to perform manicures, massages, and hairdressing. Bust of Nefertiti.

1200 B.C.
The Minoans and Mycenaeans of Greece are large producers of perfumed oil used on clothing to leave linens soft. The *Iliad* mentions the use of "slightly oiled shirts" for maidens and youth.

1000 B.C.
Tyrian dye, a purple-red pigment made from the gland of the murex shellfish, is produced in the Aegean. Its extraction is so expensive that only Greek nobility are permitted to wear the imperial purple. The dye is used as a pigment for wall paintings, as a dye for clothing, and as a rouge when mixed with chalk. Saffron, collected from the crocus flower and also used as a spice, produces an orange dye.

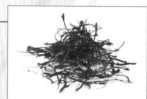

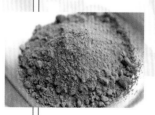

60 B.C.
Cleopatra's favorite perfume is cyprinum, a heavy scent made from the flowers of henna.

A.D. 100
The British grind cosmetic powders in small pestle and mortar sets, and use metal tweezers and toothpicks.

1000

Women of India accentuate the eyes with collyrium, a black liquid used as an early eyeliner. In India, Persia, Egypt, and much of the ancient world, lining the eyes was a form of protection against the so-called "evil eye." Temple sculpture in Khajuraho, India.

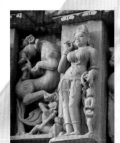

1096

The Crusading knights of Europe bring back cosmetics, perfumes, and recipes. A wide variety of beauty products are now available to women.

1200

The Arabian influence makes beauty-enhancing dyes, face cream, and lotion popular in Europe. Since the Crusades make the political climate unfavorable for direct trade, Jewish traders import spices and aromatics from the Muslim markets.

1460

John Russell's *Book of Nurture* details the methods of bathing his master, popularizing bathing in Europe. The procedure involves five or six sponges for feet and body, fresh herbs mixed in the water, and a sheet to cover the tub.

1533

Catherine de Medici marries Henry II of France and brings her personal perfumer from Italy to Paris. This launches the perfume industry in France.

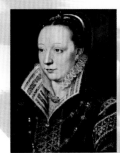

1558

The House of Tudor and the reign of Elizabeth I bring prosperity and trade with the founding of the East India Company. Most court women use cosmetics. Cosmetics are uncommon with ordinary people.

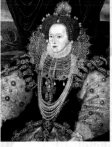
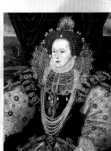

Product Development
TIMELINE
A.D. 1600. to A.D. 1800

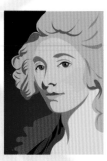

1600
Women prepare their own potions and ointments with natural ingredients passed down from family recipes.

1650
The pink and white complexion is favored in England. It is achieved with ceruse (white lead) and rouge imported from Venice.

1656
The French Guild of Glovers and Perfume Makers is established, and new scents flood the market. The Puritans object to the use of scents and beauty aids, associating them with the devil.

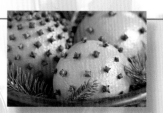

1682
Mary Doggett's *Book of Recipes* details the preparation of pomanders and sweet bags. These bags are used in the home and hang next to dress skirts to freshen them with a fragrant scent, since fine fabrics like wool and velvet were rarely laundered.

1690
John Evelyn writes *The Fop-Dictionary* and reports the use of cork pads in the mouth as a means of plumping out the cheeks, especially with women who are conscious about the loss of their teeth.

1700

Native Americans use berries to redden the cheeks and grease to smooth the hair. Some of their preparations, known as Indian Medicine, become popular.

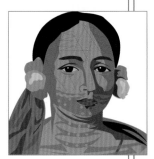

1714

Johann Maria Farina is the Cologne perfume maker primarily responsible for establishing Eau-de-Cologne as a brand.

1775

The *Toilet of Flora* written by Buc'hoz is a source for many homemade beauty treatments. Natural recipes continue to be quoted in publications to this day.

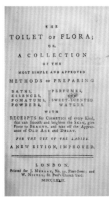

The Houbigant perfume house is founded and becomes a favorite in France, England, and Russia. Marie Antoinette and Napoleon wear their scents.

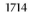

1800

Recipes for cosmetics are published in the United States.

Product Development
TIMELINE
A.D. 1814 to A.D. 1870

1814
T. W. Dyott imports cosmetics and manufactures a line of products including cold cream, skin lotion, hair powder, and pomatum. Balm of Iberia is their signature skin-perfecting product.

1834
Eugene Rimmel opens a perfumery in London and establishes the House of Rimmel. The Rimmel family would go on to produce other cosmetic products, mascara being one of their most successful. The word *rimmel* is synonymous with the word mascara in several languages.

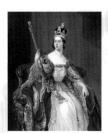

1837
Britain's Queen Victoria brings modesty and a restraint in the use of face paints. The Victorian period promotes cleanliness, grooming, and the use of lighter toilette water as a fragrance.

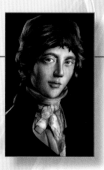

1840
A publishing boom creates more publications on beauty and fashion. Men in America discard their wigs and embrace a new understated appearance.

The first solid blushers are presented in a compact.

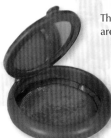
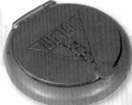

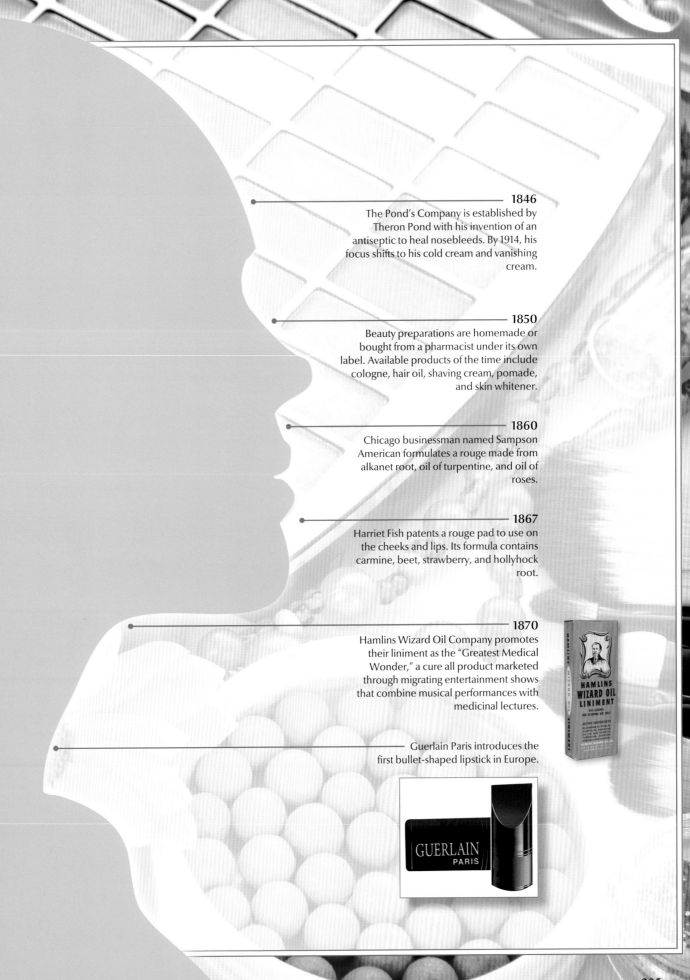

1846

The Pond's Company is established by Theron Pond with his invention of an antiseptic to heal nosebleeds. By 1914, his focus shifts to his cold cream and vanishing cream.

1850

Beauty preparations are homemade or bought from a pharmacist under its own label. Available products of the time include cologne, hair oil, shaving cream, pomade, and skin whitener.

1860

Chicago businessman named Sampson American formulates a rouge made from alkanet root, oil of turpentine, and oil of roses.

1867

Harriet Fish patents a rouge pad to use on the cheeks and lips. Its formula contains carmine, beet, strawberry, and hollyhock root.

1870

Hamlins Wizard Oil Company promotes their liniment as the "Greatest Medical Wonder," a cure all product marketed through migrating entertainment shows that combine musical performances with medicinal lectures.

Guerlain Paris introduces the first bullet-shaped lipstick in Europe.

Product Development
TIMELINE
A.D. 1872. to A.D. 1898

1872
Harper's Bazaar publishes an article on virtue and moral values, describing the benefits of plain soap and clean living.

1877
Laird's Bloom of Youth, a skin lightener containing poisonous lead, kills many women before being removed from the market.

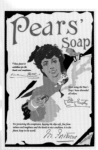

1880
Actress Lillie Langtry appears in advertisements for Hunter's Invisible Face Powder and Pears Soap.

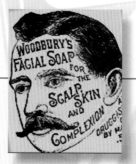

Woodbury's complexion soap is developed as a cure for skin diseases and later marketed as a beauty aid.

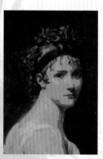

1886
Harriet Hubbard Ayer markets Recamier Cream and is one of the first women to create a cosmetics manufacturing industry in the United States. Portrait of Madam Recamier.

1888

Deodorant is invented and trademarked under the name Mum.

1889

Aimé Guerlain creates Jicky, a departure from flowery Victorian scents to a sandalwood-based scent.

1890

Lyon's Manufacturing Co. creates Hagan's Magnolia Balm, a skin lightener for African Americans.

1893

Henry Schnurman develops face bleach and hair straighteners for the African American community under the brand name Hartona.

1898

Thomas Beard Crane develops Wonderful Face Bleach.

Product Development
TIMELINE
A.D. 1900 to A.D. 1919

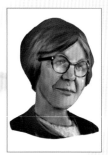

1900
Annie Turnbo Malone produces a hair treatment for African Americans called Wonderful Hair Grower and sells it door to door. In 1906, she registers it under the name Poro.

Rilas Gathright manufactures a magnetic comb, Ozono hair preparations, deodorant, and Imperial Whitener, and sells them through mail order newspaper ads.

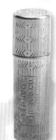

1903
Lip Ivo produces the first clear lip balm and gloss.

1904
François Coty, credited with the founding of the modern fragrance industry, creates Coty in Paris.

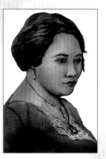

1905
Madame C. J. Walker develops a technique for pressing hair with light oil and a heated comb.

Anthony Overton introduces High-Brown face powder for African Americans.

1906
Charles Nestle invents the permanent wave.

1907
Eugene Schueller invents synthetic hair dye. This marks the beginning of L'Oréal.

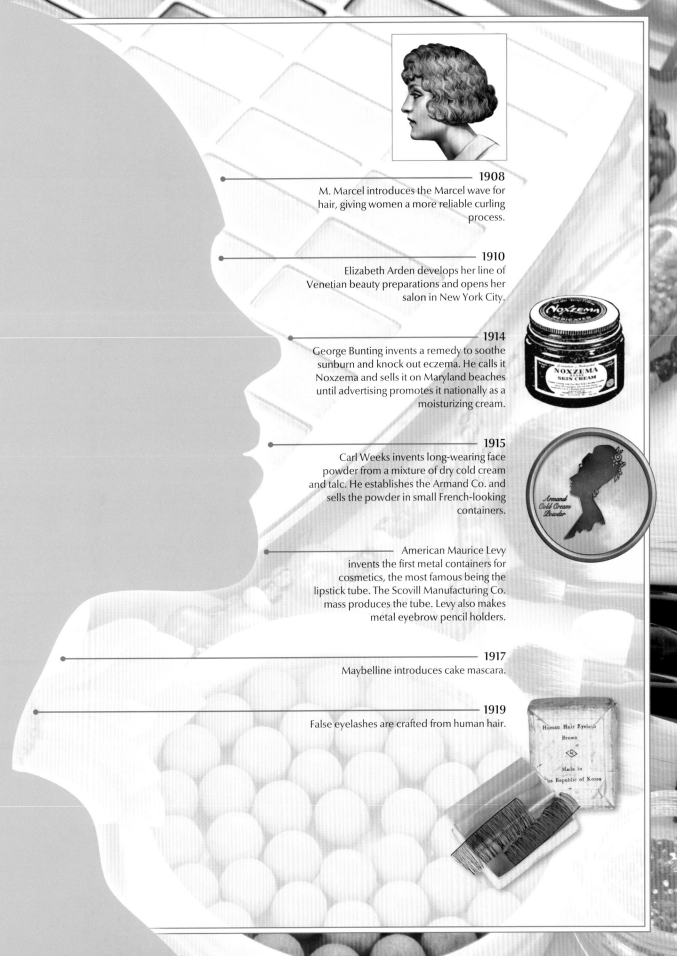

1908

M. Marcel introduces the Marcel wave for hair, giving women a more reliable curling process.

1910

Elizabeth Arden develops her line of Venetian beauty preparations and opens her salon in New York City.

1914

George Bunting invents a remedy to soothe sunburn and knock out eczema. He calls it Noxzema and sells it on Maryland beaches until advertising promotes it nationally as a moisturizing cream.

1915

Carl Weeks invents long-wearing face powder from a mixture of dry cold cream and talc. He establishes the Armand Co. and sells the powder in small French-looking containers.

American Maurice Levy invents the first metal containers for cosmetics, the most famous being the lipstick tube. The Scovill Manufacturing Co. mass produces the tube. Levy also makes metal eyebrow pencil holders.

1917

Maybelline introduces cake mascara.

1919

False eyelashes are crafted from human hair.

Product Development
TIMELINE
A.D. 1920 to A.D. 1928

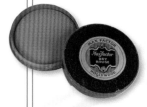

The first patent for
faint pink nail polish is granted.

1920

Max Factor introduces Society Makeup, a line
of products for everyday use. His cosmetics are
distributed nationally by 1927.

The eyebrow pencil
rises in popularity with the addition
of hydrogenated cottonseed oil to
the formula, which makes the color
glide on easily.

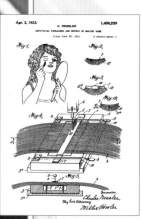

1921

Charles Nessler invents artificial
eyelashes and a manufacturing
process for them. Artificial Eyelashes
and Method of Making Same
patent, no. 1,450,259. C. Nessler, 1923.

Ernest Beaux invents the first
synthetic fragrance, Chanel No. 5.

1922

Chicago based J. E. McBrady markets a line of
"specialties for brown skin people" sold only
through agents.

1923
Kurlash, the first eyelash
curling device, is invented.

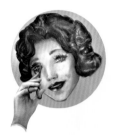

James Bruce Mason Jr.
patents the first swivel lipstick mechanism.
Toilet Article patent, no. 1,470,994. J. B.
Mason Jr., 1922.

1924
Cutex brand sells pink and
rose-colored nail polish.

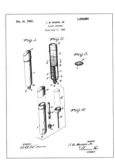

1925
Tattoo brand cosmetics and
Laleek Longlash sell mascara in a cream
made from tinted Vaseline.

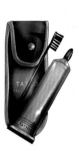

1928
Marjorie Joyner invents
the permanent wave machine and becomes
the first African American woman to receive
a patent. Permanent Waving Machine
patent, no. 1,693,515. M. S. Joyner, 1928.

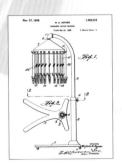

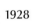

Product Development
TIMELINE
A.D. 1930 to A.D. 1958

1930
Warner's introduces cup sizes for brassieres.

Tre-Jur compacts
and Outdoor Girl powder are popular
products made in factories as private labels,
not by at-home self manufacturing. Many
start-up companies are established this way,
increasing the number of niche brands on the
market.

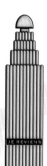

1932
House of Worth, a renowned clothing
manufacturer, creates Je Reviens fragrances.

Charles Revson,
his brother Joseph, and chemist Charles
Lachman establish the Revlon company with
the production of opaque nail polish.

1935
Tangee advertises a lipstick made with bromo-
acid that changes colors to blend naturally
with the lips. It encourages young girls to wear
natural looking makeup.

1936
Tattoo lipstick advertises a staining lipstick that
is paste free and indelible.

L'Oréal founder
Eugene Schueller invents sunscreen.

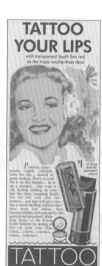

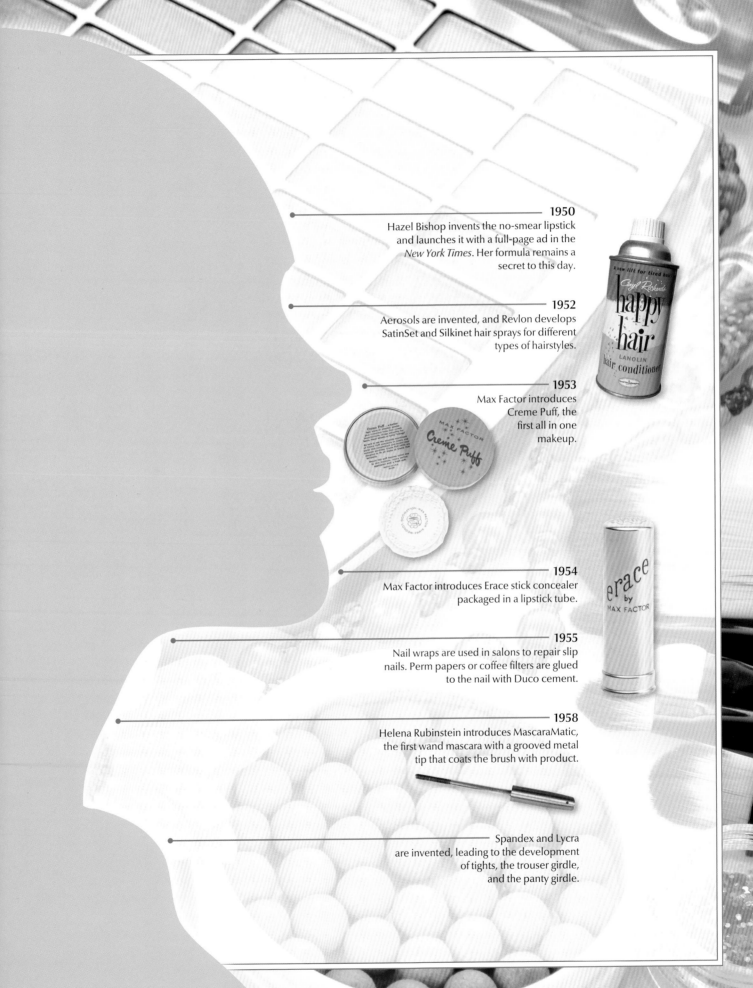

1950
Hazel Bishop invents the no-smear lipstick and launches it with a full-page ad in the *New York Times*. Her formula remains a secret to this day.

1952
Aerosols are invented, and Revlon develops SatinSet and Silkinet hair sprays for different types of hairstyles.

1953
Max Factor introduces Creme Puff, the first all in one makeup.

1954
Max Factor introduces Erace stick concealer packaged in a lipstick tube.

1955
Nail wraps are used in salons to repair slip nails. Perm papers or coffee filters are glued to the nail with Duco cement.

1958
Helena Rubinstein introduces MascaraMatic, the first wand mascara with a grooved metal tip that coats the brush with product.

Spandex and Lycra are invented, leading to the development of tights, the trouser girdle, and the panty girdle.

Product Development
TIMELINE
A.D. 1962 to A.D. 1979

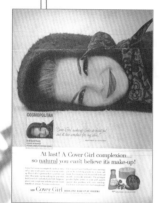

1962

CoverGirl cosmetics is introduced and promotes a young, fresh face.

1963

Flex introduces the first corrective shampoo with protein and the first anti-dandruff formula ZP11.

1965

Flori Roberts creates the first makeup range for black-skinned women.

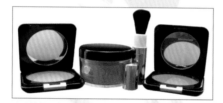

1968

Revlon introduces Eterna '27', the first cosmetic cream with an estrogen derivative called Progenitin used to keep skin hydrated and less prone to wrinkles.

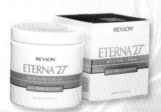

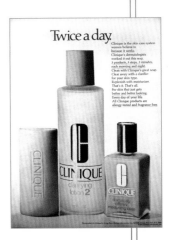

Clinique launches
with a simple line of seven products
used as a beauty prescription
for healthy skin.

1974

Sun In is a popular spray-in hair lightener
that lightens and brightens hair from brown
to blonde.

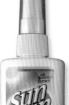
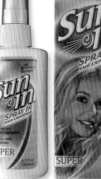

1975

Chanel introduces their first makeup line
with a collection of twenty-six lip colors.

1976

Bare Escentuals appears and promotes its
line of mineral makeup.

1979

Prescriptives is introduced with more than
170 shades and nine foundation formulas,
and delivers an exact color match to one's
natural skin tone.

PRESCRIPTIVES

Product Development
TIMELINE
A.D. 1984 to A.D. 2009

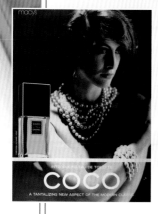

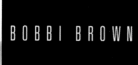

1984

Chanel introduces the Coco fragrance, a heavier scent suited to the excess of the time.

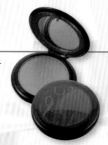

Guerlain introduces the first bronzing powder with its Terracota line.

1986

Lancome introduces Niosome, the first cream to contain liposomes that are believed to reduce wrinkles.

1991

Makeup artist Bobbi Brown launches her cosmetics line called Bobbi Brown Essentials with ten lipsticks and a philosophy that women "want to look and feel like themselves, only prettier and more confident."

1992

Yves Saint Laurent launches his famous Touché Éclat highlighter and eye brightener, an essential in many women's handbags.

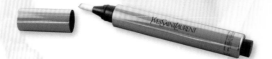

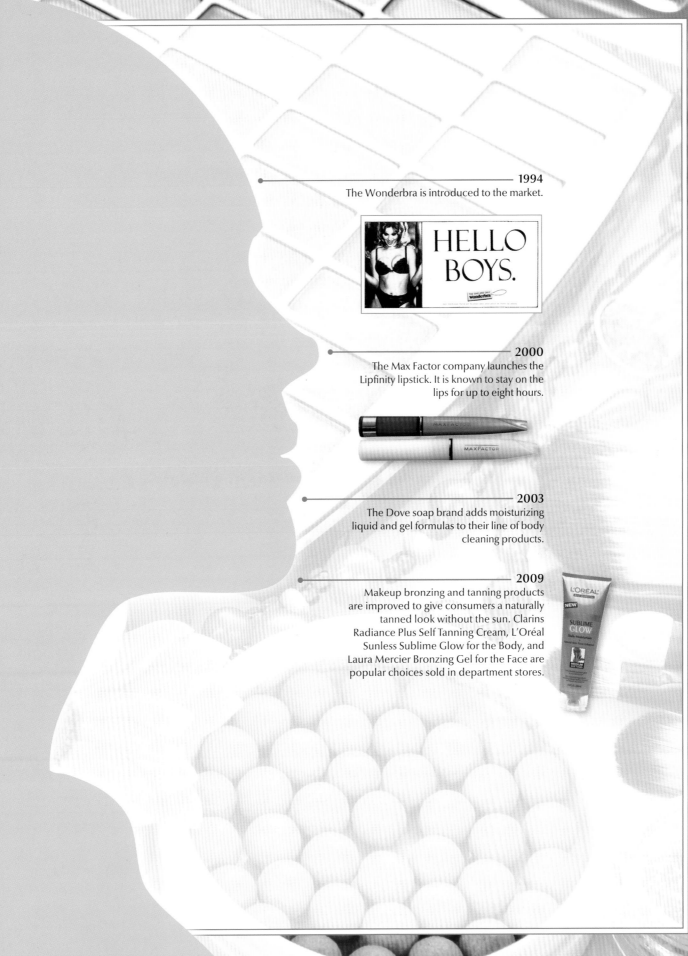

1994

The Wonderbra is introduced to the market.

HELLO
BOYS.

2000

The Max Factor company launches the Lipfinity lipstick. It is known to stay on the lips for up to eight hours.

2003

The Dove soap brand adds moisturizing liquid and gel formulas to their line of body cleaning products.

2009

Makeup bronzing and tanning products are improved to give consumers a naturally tanned look without the sun. Clarins Radiance Plus Self Tanning Cream, L'Oréal Sunless Sublime Glow for the Body, and Laura Mercier Bronzing Gel for the Face are popular choices sold in department stores.

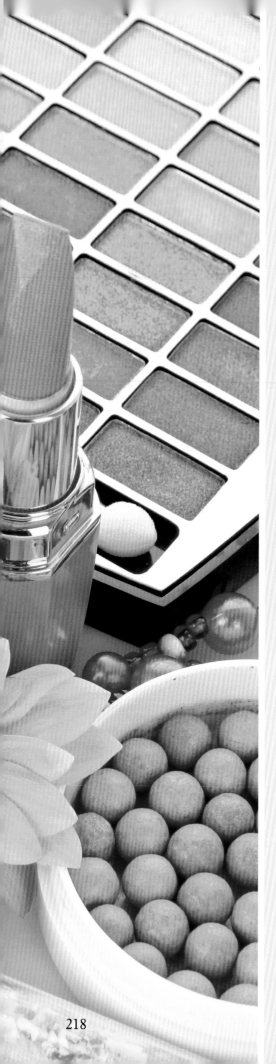

Conclusion

Why do we care so much about beauty? In the pages of this book, we have travelled through history to discover endless twists on the answer to this question. But perhaps the answer was summed up most succinctly by industry icon Elizabeth Arden who said it this way: "Beauty comes out of depth of living and feeling, out of character, faith, and the courage to act."

We are all endowed with some innate aspects of beauty by dint of our genetics. If we're lucky our DNA gifts us with the raw basics that define human beauty: symmetrical features, clear skin, full hair, nicely shaped and spaced teeth, height proportionate to weight, and so on. Most of us have to work at it a little, starting with skin care and makeup. I have devoted my life to this work, which I call the Traditions of Glamour. In my mind, this is joyful work. Finding your best look is fun, and it gives you confidence to face the challenges of the day. A woman (or a man, although this book is dedicated primarily to the glamour practices of women) who makes the effort and takes the time to let us see and enjoy her own unique glamour also raises the morale of the people she meets. Interacting with someone who is wonderfully groomed is an uplifting experience. In fact, for me, literally just seeing a woman on the street with a polished coif, great makeup, and a flattering dress and shoe—like getting a glimpse of a man in a great suit with a sharp haircut—makes my day. It does take a little effort, but making that effort literally changes your life. And doing so touches the world of everyone around you.

Of course in every generation there is a counter-movement that protests against the crimping, primping, plucking, blushing, and glossing. This counter-movement, from pious Puritans to New Age, all natural, wash-and-wear advocates, always offers the same objection: tending to our appearance is vanity, artificial, and, even worse, superficial. My work continually proves to me that just the opposite is true. The waggish and very stylish Oscar Wilde wrote that only superficial people do not judge others based on appearances. His opinion was confirmed more than a century later by Malcolm Gladwell's best-selling book, *Blink*, which examined in sociological terms how we assess others in the twinkling of an eye. People who are perceived as beautiful and glamorous wield tremendous power. Today it's called "looks-ism," but this has always been the case. Feeling groomed and well cared for is a daily mood booster, inspiring us to be our best when we look our best.

Glamour is the art and science of optimizing the gorgeousness that's in your own DNA—perhaps hidden, waiting to be revealed. Glamorous women everywhere inspire my work, starting with my own family when I was growing up in Argentina. My earliest memories of my grandmother are of a strong woman who would not leave her house without perfect hair, flawless makeup, and stunning red lipstick. Those memories are still with me every day and serve as the guiding beacon that helps invent and inspire my cosmetic line. And while it might be fair to say that I am like a mad scientist obsessed by the quest for the perfect red lipstick, what interests me even more is why a woman wants it, and how I can help her find the most perfect one that brings out the best in her.

I work in the cosmetics business, right in the heart of the entertainment industry. One of my retail locations is situated a few blocks from Warner Brothers Studios, where hundreds of the entertainment industry's most iconic films (as well as musical recordings and television shows) have been produced for many decades. Many of my clients are professional makeup artists for this industry. Los Angeles, like countless places around the globe, is filled with people who are dedicated to making themselves more beautiful— many are performers, but many more are not. This is the backdrop for my work.

Since I am a historian as well as a cosmetics formulator and designer, you might think that I am someone who is interested only in the past. But as this book demonstrates, my passion goes beyond just history. My work resonates with the present and future, rooted deeply in the Traditions of Glamour, and how contemporary glamour is always evolving while remaining coherent to classical ideas.

History shows us that women have lined their eyes, painted their lips, powdered their cheeks, and perfumed their skin and hair for centuries as a norm in order to attract a mate, and to communicate familial affiliation and social status. More importantly, doing so is a way in which we assert our power as women.

What is beautiful? The definition fluctuates, yet returns to center, as a pendulum swings. We are drawn to notions of orderliness, which underlie our most deeply held definitions of beauty. Mathematicians, philosophers, artists, and designers throughout history have referred to the golden mean or the golden ratio as an attribute of beauty. The Greeks defined this ratio as the desirable middle between two extremes and, remarkably, you don't need to know math to understand this concept. In fact, some perception of the golden mean seems to be embedded in our DNA. The early practitioners of makeup artistry used these same ratios to craft the faces of the most iconic actresses in the world, the very ones that started the reign of the Hollywood beauty queen.

Tastes change from generation to generation and across ethnic groups from around the world, creating multiple interpretations and expressions of the golden mean. In general, throughout history we have appreciated the look of large eyes, which are trusting and child-like, and a straight nose—a glimpse of Egyptian, Greek, and Roman statuary confirms this. Today's standard of facial beauty favors a wide mouth and large lips, characteristics the rigorous Athenians and Victorians might have found too overtly sensual. But our basic standard of facial beauty in particular still stays loosely in keeping with the golden ratio.

During particularly difficult times in history, making your hair, skin, and body pleasing to yourself and others was seen as an act of optimism—sometimes even an act of defiance and bravery, as it was for American, British, and French women during WWII, when wearing red lipstick sent a message of fearless support to the Allied Forces. It said, simply, "We refuse to give up." Glamour in this sense is a statement of self-worth and value. This is true at any age, size, and shape—as senior "glamourista" Iris Apfel's recent documentary, *Iris*, reminds us.

Exploring this and more has been the joy of researching and creating this book. The photos of vintage cosmetics are from my own personal collection, to which I am always adding, in my search for the next treasure to bring back from the past. I am convinced that when we pencil our lash-line and redden our lips, we are connecting with human beings who did the same thousands of years ago. I hope you enjoy reminiscing with my book as much as I have enjoyed the journey of bringing it to you. And I hope that you continue to inspire yourself and those around you with the Traditions of Glamour.

Glossary of Common Ingredients

Alkanet: Red dye obtained from a root of the Dyers Bugloss plant. Used to tint lip salve, rouge, and perfume.

Almond Nut: Used for its oil. The oil is extracted and blended with flowers to obtain the flower's scent. Added to bath water and used as a skin softener.

Aloe: A succulent plant that originated in Africa, well known as a skin soother. During the Middle Ages in Britain, it was available as a black, powdered, or dried sap.

Alum: Known for its drying qualities, a crystalline solid used as a fixative for dyes in early hair-dye recipes. Also used in stick form to stop bleeding caused by shaving cuts.

Ambergris: A natural substance produced by the sperm whale, used as a fixative ingredient in the manufacture of perfume. Due to cost and environmental restrictions on this product, synthetic versions are used in modern perfumery.

Annatto: A reddish-yellow dye extracted from the seeds of this tropical tree used as a cosmetics colorant. The tree is also called the lipstick tree.

Antimony: A mineral with a dark gray metallic finish used since pre-historic times in the preparation of kohl. Used as a cosmetic to darken the eyelids and eyebrows.

Arabic Gum: Gum resin used in cosmetics.

Arrowroot: White powder extracted from this plant is used as a base for body powder. Also used as a thickener in cooking.

Balm: Lemon-scented perennial plant from Britain used in historical perfumery.

Balsam: Small tree that produces a resinous gum.

Bay: Small evergreen shrub used in early bathing recipes for its resin scent.

Bear's Grease: An ingredient extracted from the fat of bears used since the 1600s to make early cream and rouge. Also a popular hair pomade for men during the Victorian period.

Beeswax: Natural wax produced by bees and used as an emulsifier in cosmetics.

Behen Oil: Oil derived from the nuts of the Moringa or horseradish tree. It was used by the Egyptians in perfume recipes because of its ability to remain fresh during long periods of storage.

Borax: Household cleanser that dissolves grease and softens water. Used in creams as a preservative and as a saponifier to convert fats into soap.

Carmine: Red pigment obtained from the dried bodies of the female cochineal insect. Used as a colorant for cosmetics and artists' paints.

Castor Oil: Oil from the castor bean used in lipstick and moisturizer.

Cassia: Bark with a subtle taste of cinnamon. Used in perfumes for thousands of years. Referred to in the Bible as part of the anointing oil of the Jews.

Ceruse: White lead pigment produced by a chemical reaction caused by vinegar on thin sheets of lead. The resulting white "bloom" was scraped off and used on the face to whiten the complexion. This poisonous product killed many society women and ruined the complexion of others.

Cinnabar: Tree resin known as dragon's blood used as a cosmetics colorant.

Civet: Animal extract produced in the genital region of the civet cat used in perfumery to add warmth and depth to other scents.

Coriander: Seed with an orange-like scent introduced to Britain by the Romans and used in perfumery during the fifteenth, sixteenth, and seventeenth centuries.

Crocus/Saffron: Long red stigmas of the crocus collected in autumn for use in dyes and perfume. Used by the Romans as a hair dye, eye shadow, and fabric dye. It yields a strong yellowish gold tint.

Cuttlefish: Squid-like cephalopod marine mollusk of the genus Sepia whose skeleton was ground and used as an additive in toothpowders. Believed to have been used in musky perfumes by the Romans.

Cyperus: A violet-scented plant related to the papyrus plant used in early perfume.

Face Pack: A thick paste worn for long periods to improve the skin. Its origins are traced back to Roman times.

Frankincense: Resin used in incense and perfume and as a fumigant. The lampblack produced when burning this resin was used as eyeliner. Most frankincense comes from Somalia and Arabia. Used by the Egyptians in cosmetic recipes as an oil to keep the skin looking young.

French Chalk: Finely ground magnesium silicate used to powder the face.

Fucus: Dye of the lichen plant created by fermenting it with alkali. Produces a purple/red color that dissipates in sunlight. Used by Greeks and Romans as an inexpensive rouge.

Gillyflower: A clove scented flower used to infuse wine and perfume. Used heavily in Tudor perfumes.

Hair Powder: Powder made from ground animal bone, starch, and flour, scented with cypress civet and musk. Used in the eighteenth century with pomade to style white wigs.

Henna: A reddish-orange dye extracted from the leaves and flowers of this plant. Used as a dye for cosmetics and for coloring fabrics. Its flowers were used to make Camphire, Cleopatra's favorite fragrance. Used as a hair dye in the Medieval period. Used in Egypt to stain the skin.

Kaolin: White Chinese clay used in powders and face masks.

Kohl: A black powder, such as powdered antimony sulfide or lampblack, produced by the burning of resin. Used by women in Egypt and Arabia as a cosmetic to darken the eyelids and eyebrows.

Lampblack: Almost pure carbon obtained by burning resin or some other substance. Provides a black pigment for eye paint or ink.

Lanolin: Oil extracted from sheep's wool used in cosmetics as a moisturizer for the skin.

Lye: A strong caustic alkaline solution of potassium salts used in soap making by percolating rainwater through hardwood ashes.

Mineral Oil: A by-product of petroleum used in cosmetics.

Musk: Substance produced by the musk gland of a mature male musk deer. Used to infuse fragrances and provide fixative qualities to the scent. Fabrication today is of synthetic origin because most countries prohibit the trading of natural musk in order to protect the endangered deer.

Olive Oil: Oil extracted from the olive fruit and used in cooking and soap. During the Medieval and Tudor periods, it was used in ointments to moisturize the skin.

Orris Root: Plant root used to make violet-scented skin powders. Also used in early toothpowder recipes.

Paraffin: Waxy substance derived from petroleum and used as a thickener for creams.

Pomander: A wooden ball or other round object perfumed with scented waxes to obscure bad odors. It was kept where clothing was stored or worn on girdles.

Quicklime: Calcium oxide obtained by heating limestone. A white caustic alkaline substance used in bleaching powder, cement, and plaster.

Rose: Grown as early as 4000 years ago, it is one of the oldest plants cultivated by man. Used in perfume, ointment, and rose water.

Rouge: Red powder or cream for the lips and cheeks, usually made with ochre, alkanet, cochineal, or Brazil wood. It was applied as a powder or salve and also from a cloth or pad of wool impregnated with strong dye. Rouge has been thought to be the most universal cosmetic throughout history.

Spanish Leather: A highly perfumed leather square or dyed leather traded throughout Europe and used from the Tudor period forward. The red dyed leather was dampened and used as rouge.

Tansy: Bitter herb used to make skin washer and toners during the 1500s and 1600s.

Unguent: Ointment with a high fat content used as a scented salve in a liquid or solid state.

Vermillion: A water-insoluble pigment used as rouge. Worn by the Greeks, Romans, and Chinese even though it was found to be a highly dangerous pigment. Also known as red mercuric sulfide and commonly used in artist pigments.

Bibliography

Angeloglou, Maggie. *A History of Makeup*. London: The Macmillan Company, 1970.

Antoine Dariaux, Genevieve. *A Guide to Elegance: For Every Woman Who Wants to be Well and Properly Dressed on All Occasions*. United Kingdom: HarperCollins Publishers UK, 2003.

Batchelor, Bob. *The 2000s: American Pop Culture Through History*. Westport, CT: Greenwood Press, 2009.

Bjork, Angela and Daniela Turudich. *Vintage Face: Period Looks from the 20s, 30s, 40s, & 50s*. California: Streamline Press, 2001.

Chahine, Nathalie, et al. *Beauty: The Twentieth Century*. New York: Universe Publishing, 2000.

Cohen Ragas, Meg and Karen Kozlowski. *Read My Lips: A Cultural History of Lipstick*. San Francisco: Chronicle Books, 1998.

Durkee, Cutler, ed. *People: Celebrate the '70s! Stars, Fads and Fashions from an Amazing Decade*. New York: People Books, Time Inc., 2009.

Eco, Umberto, ed. *History of Beauty*. New York: Rizzoli International Publications, Inc., 2004.

Feinstein, Stephen. *The 1980s: From Ronald Reagan to MTV*. Berkeley Heights, NJ: Enslow Publishers, Inc., 2006.

Gavenas, Mary Lisa. *Color Stories: Behind the Scenes of America's Billion-Dollar Beauty Industry*. New York: Simon & Schuster, 2002.

Gunn, Fenja. *The Artificial Face: A History of Cosmetics*. New York: Hippocrene Books, 1983.

Mulvey, Kate and Melissa Richards. *Decades of Beauty: The Changing Image of Women 1890s to 1990s*. New York: Octopus Publishing Group LTD., 1998.

Pallingston, Jessica. *Lipstick: A Celebration of the World's Favorite Cosmetic*. New York: St. Martin's Press, 1999.

Peiss, Kathy. *Hope in a Jar: The Making of America's Beauty Culture*. New York: Henry Holt and Company Inc., 1999.

Phillips, M. C. *Skin Deep: The Truth About Beauty Aids*. New York: The Vanguard Press, 1934.

Pointer, Sally. *The Artifice of Beauty: A History and Practical Guide to Perfumes and Cosmetics*. United Kingdom: Sutton Publishing, 2005.

Riordan, Teresa. *Inventing Beauty: A History of the Innovations That Have Made Us Beautiful*. New York: Broadway Books, 2004.

Rustenholz, Alain. *Make Up*. London: Hachette Illustrated UK, 2003.

Stewart, Gail B. *The 1970s: A Cultural History of the United States Through the Decades*. San Diego, CA: Lucent Books, Inc., 1999.

Swinfield, Rosemarie. *Period Makeup for the Stage*. Cincinnati: Betterway Books, 1997.

Time-Life Books. *The Digital Decade: The 90s*. New York: Bishop Books, 2000.

Vail, Gilbert Miller. *A History of Cosmetics in America*. New York: The Toilet Goods Association, Inc., 1947.

Verrill, A. Hyatt. *Perfumes and Spices*. Massachusetts: L. C. Page & Company, 1940.

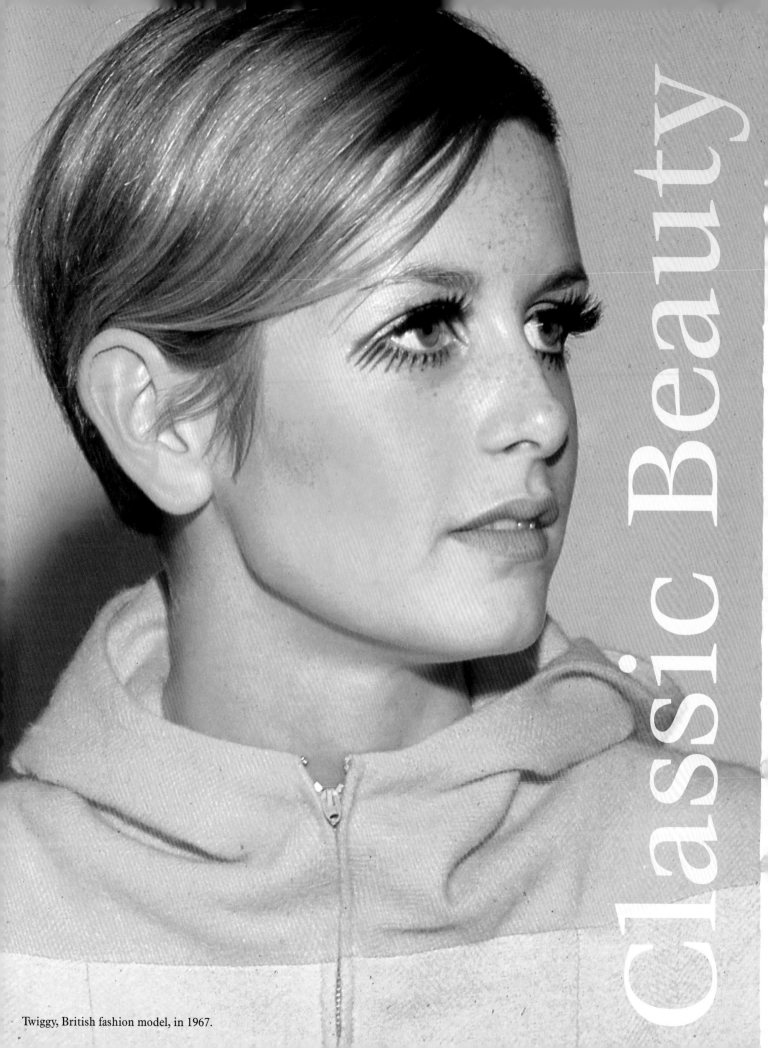

Classic Beauty

Twiggy, British fashion model, in 1967.

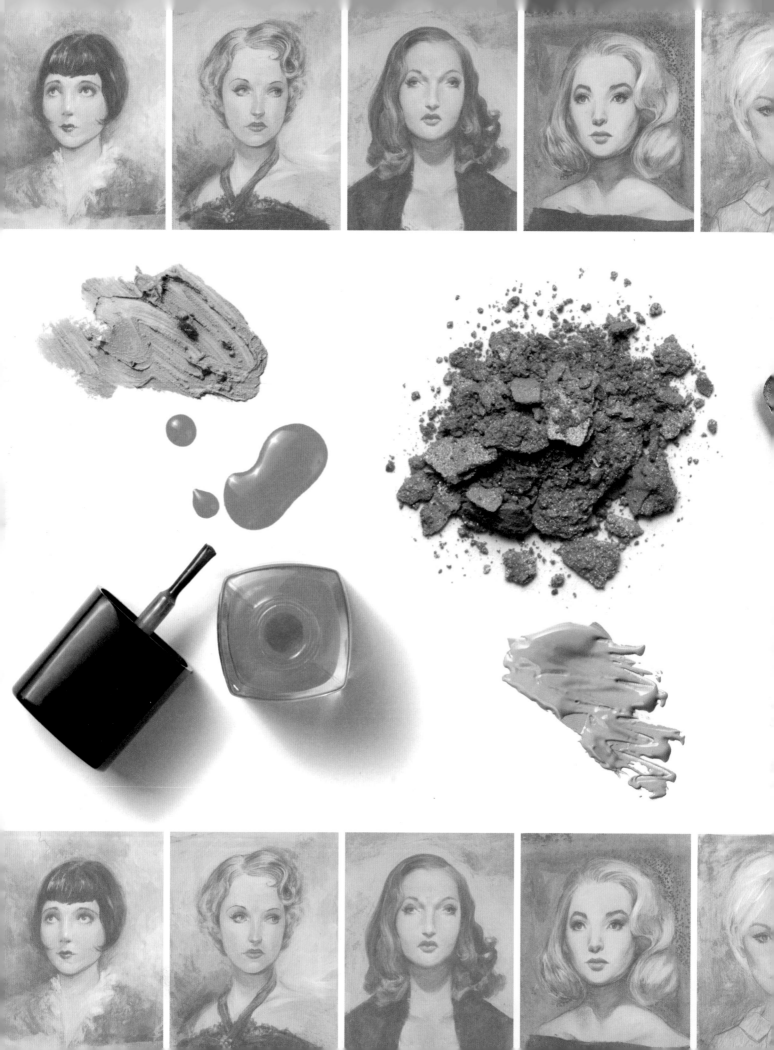